Vascular access

SIMPLIFIED

Edited by

Alun H Davies & Christopher P Gibbons

SECOND EDITION

tfm Publishing Limited, Castle Hill Barns, Harley, Nr Shrewsbury, SY5 6LX, UK. Tel: +44 (0)1952 510061; Fax: +44 (0)1952 510192 E-mail: nikki@tfmpublishing.com; Web site: www.tfmpublishing.com

Design & Typesetting: Nikki Bramhill, tfm publishing Ltd.
Second Edition: © 2007

ISBN: 978 1 903378 52 6

Printed by Gutenberg Press Ltd., Gudja Road, Tarxien, PLA 19, Malta. Tel: +356 21897037; Fax: +356 21800069.

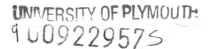

Contents

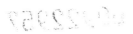

Contributors

Alison J Armitage MB ChB MRCP MD Senior Registrar in Nephrology, Southmead Hospital, Bristol, UK

Ali Bakran FRCS (Eng) FRCS (Edin) Consultant Vascular & Transplant Surgeon, Royal Liverpool University Hospital, Liverpool, UK

Pierre Bourquelot MD Vascular Access Surgeon, Vascular Access Department, Clinique Jouvenet, Paris, France

Edwina Brown DM FRCP Consultant Nephrologist, West London Renal and Transplant Centre, Hammersmith Hospital, London, UK

Peter WG Brown BSc FRCS FRCR Consultant Radiologist, Sheffield Teaching Hospitals NHS Trust, Sheffield, UK

Peter Choi MA MB PhD MRCP Consultant Nephrologist, West London Renal and Transplant Centre, Hammersmith Hospital, London, UK

Alison J Cornall RN BA (Hons) MSc Vascular Access Nurse Specialist, Churchill Hospital, Oxford, UK

Alun H Davies MA DM FRCS Reader in Surgery and Consultant Surgeon, Imperial College School of Medicine, Charing Cross Hospital, London, UK

Paula A Davies RN Vascular Access Nurse Specialist, Morriston Hospital, Swansea, UK

Stephen D'Souza MB ChB FRCP FRCR Consultant Interventional Radiologist, Lancashire Teaching Hospitals, Lancashire, UK

Andrew H Frankel BSc MB BS MD FRCP Consultant Nephrologist, West London Renal and Transplant Centre, Hammersmith Hospital, London, UK

Christopher P Gibbons MA DPhil MCh FRCS Consultant Surgeon, Morriston Hospital, Swansea, UK

George Hamilton MD FRCS Professor of Vascular Surgery, Royal Free Hampstead NHS Trust, Royal Free & University College School of Medicine, London, UK

David C Mitchell MA MB MS FRCS Consultant Vascular & Transplant Surgeon, Southmead Hospital, Bristol, UK

Andrew T Raftery BSc MD FRCS Consultant Surgeon, Sheffield Kidney Institute, Northern General Hospital, Sheffield, UK

Nung Rudarakanchana PhD MRCS Senior House Officer, Charing Cross Hospital, London, UK

Badri M Shrestha BSc MS MPhil FRCS Consultant Surgeon, Sheffield Kidney Institute, Northern General Hospital, Sheffield, UK

David Taube FRCP Consultant Nephrologist and Professor of Transplant Medicine, West London Renal and Transplant Centre, Hammersmith Hospital, London, UK

Charles RV Tomson MA BM BCh FRCP DM (Oxon) Consultant Nephrologist, Southmead Hospital, Bristol, UK

Janice Tsui MD MRCS Vascular Specialist Registrar, Royal Free Hampstead NHS Trust, Royal Free & University College School of Medicine, London, UK

Andrew J Williams MD FRCP Consultant Nephrologist, Morriston Hospital, Swansea, UK

Preface

The creation of access for dialysis has long been a neglected branch of surgery. Because of its origin in nephrology and the subsequent uptake by surgeons from a variety of disciplines including transplantation, urology and vascular surgery, it has tended to fall in between all of them. Nephrologists have known the importance of good access for many years. Access surgery demands skill and experience to achieve good results and avoid problems. The more difficult cases can require surgical inventiveness. It requires a multidisciplinary approach, with close co-operation between physicians, surgeons, radiologists and nurses. It is also immensely rewarding.

It is hoped that this book will appeal to all medical and paramedical professionals involved with patients requiring renal access, and will be a useful and practical guide to current practice in the creation and maintenance of dialysis access. It may be particularly useful for the increasing numbers of vascular and other surgeons who are taking on dialysis access in an expanding number of renal units.

Alun H Davies
Christopher P Gibbons
April 2007

Chapter 1

Vascular access in clinical practice

Christopher P Gibbons MA DPhil MCh FRCS

Consultant Surgeon, Morriston Hospital, Swansea, UK

Introduction

Access to the circulation is vital in many branches of medicine. In most cases a temporary route of access for delivering fluids or drugs to the venous system is all that is required. In other cases small quantities of venous or arterial blood must be withdrawn intermittently for haematological or biochemical analysis. Simple intravenous or arterial catheters are sufficient to accomplish these tasks. More specialised intravenous catheters introduced into the central veins are required for long-term intravenous feeding or for the administration of cytotoxic chemotherapy. By contrast, haemodialysis or haemofiltration requires the reliable withdrawal and return of blood to the circulation at high flow rates (preferably exceeding 300ml/min) on a regular basis.

The Scribner shunt was the first vascular access device used to allow circulation of blood from the arterial system through a dialyser to the venous system. This was used for several years but proved unreliable for long-term access because of repeated thrombosis and infection. It was also unpopular with patients because of its cumbersome extracorporeal tubing. The arteriovenous (AV) fistula, first introduced by Brescia and Cimino in 1966, involves the conversion of an accessible peripheral vein, usually in the upper limb, to a high flow vessel from which blood can be rapidly withdrawn and returned to the circulation via two needles introduced for each dialysis session. This dispensed with the need for extracorporeal tubing between dialyses and allowed greater freedom for patients undergoing chronic renal replacement therapy. However, the need for a period of maturation generally precludes the use of AV fistulae for acute dialysis. In the absence of a suitable superficial vein, prosthetic grafts run subcutaneously from an artery to a vein can be used, but they are usually reserved for secondary access because of poorer patency and greater infection rates.

The introduction of dual-lumen central venous catheters supplanted the Scribner shunt for emergency and short-term use. More recent modifications have included the incorporation of a Dacron cuff around the catheters, which enables long-term fixation in a subcutaneous tunnel and acts as a barrier to infection. Single-lumen catheters with a Dacron cuff have also proved useful for long-term intravenous feeding and drug administration.

Whilst the vast majority of vascular access procedures are performed for haemodialysis, the access surgeon may occasionally be called upon to create an AV fistula for patients requiring plasmapheresis, to insert a long-term catheter for intravenous feeding or implant an injection port for the infusion of chemotherapeutic agents.

Renal replacement therapy

Haemodialysis is the most prevalent mode of chronic renal replacement therapy and is now almost universally used for acute dialysis. Peritoneal dialysis is an effective alternative mode of therapy, which allows greater independence for some patients. Unfortunately, the effectiveness of peritoneal dialysis tends to reduce after several years because of changes that occur in the peritoneal membrane. Renal transplantation is the preferred mode of treatment for most patients as it allows a near normal lifestyle, albeit at the expense of long-term immunosuppression, but many patients will return to dialysis after irreversible acute or chronic rejection. Thus, patients with end-stage renal failure will often move from one modality of treatment to another.

When is dialysis needed?

Acute renal failure

Temporary or permanent haemodialysis via a central venous catheter is required when the kidneys fail acutely, regardless of the underlying cause.

In some patients with acute renal failure, dialysis may be deferred or avoided by careful fluid restriction, and the control of acidosis and hyperkalaemia using intravenous bicarbonate, salbutamol or insulin and glucose combined with enteral resonium. When there is anuria or severe oliguria with fluid overload, gross metabolic acidosis, hyperkalaemia and a rising serum creatinine, acute haemodialysis via a central line will be required as a matter of urgency. In some patients, particularly those with fluid overload, for instance patients with multi-organ failure in the intensive care unit, continuous techniques involving haemofiltration and/or dialysis can be performed through a double-lumen central venous catheter.

In those patients with a treatable or spontaneously recoverable renal failure, dialysis may be discontinued as urine flow returns and serum biochemistry stabilises, but some will progress to require long-term renal replacement therapy. Once it is clear that renal recovery is unlikely, permanent vascular or peritoneal access should be created as soon as possible to minimise the use of central venous lines with their attendant increased risks of systemic infection and thrombosis. Central venous catheters are associated with a relative mortality risk of 1.7 in non-diabetics and 1.54 in diabetics in comparison to autogenous AV fistulae [1]. In the US, the National Kidney Foundation - Dialysis Outcomes Quality Initiative (NKF-DOQI) guidelines recommend that less than 10% of patients should be dialysed on lines beyond three months [2].

Chronic renal failure

A third of patients with chronic end-stage renal failure present acutely or are referred within three months of the need for dialysis. Two thirds have progressive renal disease presenting with symptoms of malaise over a period of time or are discovered by routine biochemical tests during the investigation of hypertension, proteinuria or other medical problems. It is recommended by the UK Renal Association that patients should be referred to a nephrologist when the serum creatinine is 150-200µmol/l [3]. The serum biochemistry and especially the creatinine clearance of such patients can then be monitored as an outpatient so that the need for dialysis may be anticipated. The actual start of dialysis may be primarily dependent on symptoms (e.g. malaise, nausea, anorexia, weight loss, itching), but is sometimes precipitated by an acute deterioration in biochemistry during intercurrent illness or by dehydration.

Nevertheless, dialysis is usually required at a plasma creatinine of 500-1500μmol/l or when the creatinine clearance falls much below 14ml/minute. Plotting biochemical indices of renal function, such as creatinine clearance, for each patient may give an approximate date at which dialysis is likely to be necessary (see Chapter 2). When the start of dialysis can be anticipated, permanent vascular access should be created well in advance to allow for maturation of an AV fistula or for further procedures in the event of failure of the initial access. Peritoneal dialysis catheters should be inserted between 2-4 weeks from the anticipated date of onset of dialysis.

Guidelines for vascular access timing

In the US, the NKF-DOQI guidelines recommend [2]:

◆ permanent vascular access should be constructed one year in advance of the anticipated need for dialysis, when the creatinine clearance falls below 25ml/minute or the serum creatinine rises above 4mg/dl (400μmol/l);

◆ a new primary AV fistula should be allowed to mature for at least one month and preferably 3-4 months prior to cannulation;

◆ dialysis AV grafts should be placed at least 3-6 weeks prior to an anticipated need for haemodialysis in patients who are not suitable candidates for primary AV fistulae;

◆ haemodialysis catheters should not be inserted until haemodialysis is needed.

The Vascular Access Society recommendations [4] are similar, stating that the anticipated mode of dialysis should be decided upon when the GFR reaches 20-25ml/minute and that an experienced access surgeon should see the patient when the GFR is 10-15ml/minute so that suitable access can be created 6-12 months in advance of dialysis. They also emphasise the need to preserve the forearm and upper arm veins on both sides for future access, avoiding venepuncture and cannulation at these sites.

In the UK the Renal Association [3] and the Joint Working Party of the Renal Association, The Vascular Society of Great Britain and Ireland and the British Society of Interventional Radiology [5] have produced the following service standards:

◆ at least 67% of patients presenting within three months of dialysis should start haemodialysis with a usable native AV fistula;
◆ at least 80% of prevalent haemodialysis patients should be dialysed using a native AV fistula;
◆ no patient already requiring dialysis should wait more than four weeks for fistula construction including those who present late;
◆ permanent vascular access should be created if possible at least 16 weeks and preferably six months before the anticipated need for dialysis.

Unfortunately, current practice in the UK often falls short of these standards. Whereas elsewhere in Europe, especially France and Germany, patients may receive their permanent access rapidly and efficiently, at present the under-provision of vascular access services in the UK mean that at least 50% of patients start dialysis with a central line (68% in the 2005 UK Renal Registry Report) in comparison with the European average of 33% [6-8]. This also accounts for the high prevalence of patients dialysing on central lines in the UK (31%) [6]. The Dialysis Outcomes and Practice Patterns Study (DOPPS) has shown that 58% of British patients have to wait more than three months for their first access after referral in comparison with 5% in Germany and France. Delays occur at all stages of referral, so that as many as 50% of those patients known to nephrologists more than 12 months beforehand start dialysis on a central venous catheter [6].

Conclusions

Patients with renal failure should, wherever possible, be referred early to a nephrologist so that permanent access can be constructed in advance of the need for dialysis to minimise the use of central venous lines. Where patients present in acute renal failure, dialysis must begin with a central venous catheter. However, there should be early provision of permanent vascular access in the form of an AV fistula or peritoneal access as soon as renal function is deemed irreversible.

Key Summary

◆ Haemodialysis, peritoneal dialysis and renal transplantation are all parts of an integrated renal replacement therapy program.

◆ For patients presenting acutely, dialysis must start on central venous lines whilst awaiting permanent access.

◆ In patients with chronic renal failure the use of central venous catheters should be minimised by early construction of an AV fistula.

◆ For patients with chronic renal failure, early referral to a nephrologist allows the need for dialysis to be anticipated and for an AV fistula to be created and to mature prior to the onset of dialysis.

References

1. Dhingra RK, Young EW, Hulbert-Shearon TE, *et al*. Type of vascular access and mortality in U.S. hemodialysis patients. *Kidney Int* 2001; 60: 1443-51.
2. NKF-DOQI clinical practice guidelines for vascular access. National Kidney Foundation - Dialysis Outcomes Quality Initiative. *Am J Kidney Dis* 1997; 30 (4) Suppl 3: S150-S191.
3. The Renal Association. *Treatment of adults and children with renal failure. Standards and audit measures*, 3rd edition. www.renal.org.
4. Vascular Access Society Guidelines. http://www.vascularaccesssociety.com.
5. Winearls CG, Fluck R, Mitchell DC, *et al*. The organization and delivery of the vascular access service for maintenance haemodialysis patients. Report of a joint working party, 2006. http://www.vascularsociety.org.uk/Docs/VASCULAR%20ACCESS%20JOINT%20WORKING%20PARTY%20 REPORT.pdf.

6. UK Renal Registry Report 2005. UK Renal Registry, Bristol, UK. Ansell D, Feest T, Williams AJ, Winearls C, Eds. Chapter 6; The National Dialysis Access Survey - preliminary results, 2005: 87-102. http://www.renalreg.com/Report%202005/Cover _Frame 2.htm.
7. Goodkin DA, Mapes DL, Held PJ. The Dialysis Outcomes and Practice Patterns Study (DOPPS): how can we improve the care of hemodialysis patients? *Semin Dial* 2001; 14: 157-9.
8. The Kidney Alliance. *End Stage Renal Failure - A Framework for Planning and Service Delivery*. London: Munro and Forster, 2001.

Chapter 2
Indications for chronic renal access

David **Taube** FRCP

Consultant Nephrologist and Professor of Transplant Medicine

West London Renal and Transplant Centre, Hammersmith Hospital, London, UK

Introduction

The vast majority of vascular access is primarily intended for adult haemodialysis. Its indications are essentially those of end-stage renal failure, as haemodialysis will be used as the primary form of renal replacement therapy in the majority of patients. The term 'indication' is variably used and abused in medicine; for the purposes of this chapter, the chosen definitions are 'anything that suggests the proper treatment of a disease' [1] and 'a symptom which suggests a particular disease syndrome or remedial course of action' [2].

The ideal world

In an ideal world, the need and timing for vascular access should be determined by the patient's level and rate of decline of renal function, symptoms and signs.

The real world

In real life, the placement of vascular access is not only determined by these factors but is also dependent on the availability of the appropriate facilities and in many parts of the world, including the UK, whether haemodialysis is offered as a primary therapy for end-stage renal failure (ESRF). There is no point in creating an arteriovenous (AV) fistula if haemodialysis facilities are limited or non-existent. Furthermore, many patients with ESRF present too late for elective surgery so that arteriovenous access must be created as an emergency.

In some patients the development of end-stage renal failure can be very slow and insidious. The creation of arteriovenous access implies that dialysis is necessary and many patients (and sometimes their physicians) have difficulty in accepting this. As a result, access formation may be delayed or performed in a hurry if the patient's renal function suddenly declines in the setting of another intercurrent, exacerbating factor such as an infection.

This chapter deals with the 'ideal world', concentrating on the patient's degree of renal impairment, symptoms and signs, consistent with the accepted UK (Renal Association) and US (National Kidney Foundation) published standards.

An AV fistula should be created at least three months before its intended use and a prosthetic graft or other artificial device at least two weeks before it is required. Central lines can be used immediately.

In general, arteriovenous access should be planned when the glomerular filtration rate (GFR) is less than 30ml/minute and created when the GFR is less than 20ml/minute with a view to starting dialysis when the GFR is less than 15ml/minute.

Renal impairment: the level and rate of decline of renal function

Assessment of renal function in patients with renal disease

The GFR is the best measure of renal function for which a variety of methods are clinically available. These include the plasma creatinine, serum cystatin C, creatinine clearance (CrCl), formulae derived from the plasma creatinine to estimate CrCl and specific techniques using radiocontrast agents, radionuclides such as (^{51}Cr)edetate, (^{125}I) iothalamate or inulin. These specific tests of GFR are regarded as gold standards and, although clinically available, are not generally used in day-to-day practice [3]. The methods of GFR measurement, particularly those relevant to clinical practice, have been recently reviewed by Stevens *et al* [4].

Plasma creatinine

The most robust measurement of renal function is the plasma creatinine which is a simple but imperfect measurement of the GFR because creatinine concentration is affected by a variety of factors other than creatinine filtration.

In adults, the normal range of the plasma creatinine is 60-125µmol/l and it is important to understand that a sustained increase in plasma creatinine above the upper limit of the normal range may represent a 50% reduction in GFR [5].

Most creatinine is derived from skeletal muscle, but a small amount (2%) comes from the diet of meat-eating individuals. Thus patients with a small muscle mass, who do not eat meat and who may be wasting because of their ill health often have relatively 'low' or 'normal' plasma creatinines but severely impaired GFRs. This is typically the case in West London in vegetarian Indo-Asians with chronic renal impairment. Conversely, Afro-Caribbean patients, who may have a large muscle mass, may have elevated plasma creatinines but a normal GFR.

In addition to glomerular clearance, creatinine is secreted by the tubule and is also broken down in the gut by bacteria, particularly in patients with renal failure.

Progressive fractional tubular hypersecretion of creatinine occurs in renal disease and thus the plasma creatinine, creatinine clearance and predictive formulae based on plasma creatinine will overestimate the true GFR [4, 5].

Tubular secretion of creatinine can be inhibited by commonly-used drugs such as trimethoprim, cimetidine, spironolactone and amiloride, thus raising the plasma creatinine without affecting true GFR.

Creatinine clearance

This is the most commonly used test in clinical practice and if performed correctly, is a simple, cheap and repeatable measure of GFR [6]. The real disadvantage of this investigation is that the accurate collection of urine over a 24-hour period can be difficult for busy, otherwise occupied individuals. Unlike the plasma creatinine, CrCl and true GFR declines with age [3].

Prediction of creatinine clearance using formulae based on the plasma creatinine

Various formulae have been developed to predict creatinine clearance from the plasma creatinine. These take age, sex and muscle mass into account and are routinely employed in clinical practice. The most popular was that of Cockcroft and Gault [7]. More recently, a new formula [8] has been developed as part of the Modification of Diet in Renal Disease (MDRD) Study. This formula known as the MDRD Study Prediction equation or, more simply, the MDRD equation, is based on reciprocal creatinine levels, age and mass like the Cockcroft-Gault equation, but additionally includes ethnicity, and urea and albumin levels. The MDRD equation is easily implemented into routine clinical practice. It is more accurate in predicting GFR, particularly when the GFR is less than 80ml/minute, than either formal creatinine clearance or the Cockcroft-Gault equation [4, 8]. Simpler versions of the MDRD equation are also available and have been shown to be of value in predicting GFR. The MDRD equation is now used routinely throughout the UK, both in primary and secondary care and is reported by most biochemistry laboratories in conjunction with the plasma creatinine. This equation is also the basis of the classification of the different levels of GFR used to stratify patients with chronic kidney disease in the UK and US [4].

Other methods of measuring the GFR and predicting the need for dialysis

It has been recently shown that the serum cystatin C (CysC) is a useful marker of GFR, which does not rely on the plasma creatinine. CysC is a low-molecular-weight protein constantly synthesized by all nucleated cells, the rate of which is independent of age, gender, fever, nutrition or changes in body mass. No tubular secretion or endogenous degradation has been described and it would appear that the level of this molecule is an ideal way of estimating GFR. Its measurement is not yet widely available in a clinical setting but it is likely that CysC or molecules with similar properties will supersede the plasma creatinine as a marker of GFR [9, 10].

Because the plasma creatinine and urea are inaccurate predictors of GFR and the timing or adequacy of dialysis, urea kinetic modelling (UKM) has been proposed as a better marker not only for dialysis adequacy but also as a tool to determine the need for renal replacement therapy [11, 12]. This technique, which is in routine clinical use to determine dialysis adequacy, is however not commonly used predialysis despite its advocacy by the NKF [12].

Prediction of the rate of decline of renal function

It has been known for many years that the slope of the relationship between the reciprocal plasma creatinine versus time is a useful way of measuring the rate of renal failure progression in individual patients, their response to treatment and predicting when they will require renal replacement therapy [13]. However, this technique is prone to error because spontaneous breakpoints in the slope of reciprocal plasma creatinine occur in 30-50% of patients [14].

Thus the plasma creatinine, and the Cockcroft-Gault and MDRD equations are the simplest and most effective methods of predicting GFR and assessing renal function in patients with renal failure with the proviso that these techniques are likely to overestimate GFR. In the near future, GFR measurement using better markers like cystatin C will become routinely available.

Correlation of GFR and the development of uraemic symptoms and signs

There are good data which show that the extent and severity of patients' uraemic symptoms and signs are determined by and correlate with the level of GFR [12].

GFR 30-60ml/minute

It is poorly appreciated that the 'softer' symptoms of uraemia such as increased fatigue, insomnia, a bad taste in the mouth and malodorous breath, reduced exercise tolerance and depression, commonly occur at relatively high levels of GFR (60ml/minute) [15].

Fluid retention and renal osteodystrophy are common within this band of renal function.

GFR <30ml/minute

Nausea, vomiting, intractable itching, peripheral and pulmonary oedema, and impaired mental ability occur when the GFR is less than 30ml/minute.

Coma, palmar flap, pericarditis and fulminant pulmonary oedema which were the commonly-taught indications for dialysis are features of terminal uraemia and occur when the GFR is less than 5ml/minute.

Uraemic symptoms and signs are frequently ignored or overlooked by both ESRF patients and their doctors. However, patients quickly learn to recognise the symptoms of increasing renal impairment but, because they wish to postpone the inevitable need for dialysis, may under-report their symptoms. The inadequate provision of resources for the treatment of patients with ESRF, particularly in the UK, ensures that some element of dialysis rationing takes place. Thus, doctors working in hard-pressed renal units will inevitably delay the acceptance of patients for dialysis, especially those who are relatively asymptomatic.

Diabetic nephropathy and poor left ventricular function

Some patients, particularly diabetics and patients with poor left ventricular function, may require dialysis at relatively high levels of GFR.

Clinical anecdote suggests that patients with diabetic nephropathy tend to have more uraemic symptoms than non-diabetics with similar low levels of GFR. Whether this is a reflection of their other non-renal problems (especially neuropathy and retinopathy) in combination with their uraemia is uncertain. Patients with poor left ventricular function and non-salt-losing forms of renal failure are particularly prone to the consequences of fluid overload. These patients may become diuretic-resistant at relatively high levels of GFR and require early initiation of dialysis.

The timing of access formation and the initiation of dialysis

It has been generally believed that the early initiation of dialysis is associated with a better outcome, with a reduced mortality and length of hospital stay [16]. However, there are no rigorous randomised controlled clinical trials that indicate precisely when and at what level of GFR, dialysis should be initiated [16]. The NKF-DOQI guidelines suggest a GFR range between 9-14ml/minute and a KT/V <2.0 [12]. However, the literature is conflicting, as some studies have failed to demonstrate that early initiation of dialysis improves prognosis [17]. Prospective studies would require huge numbers of patients enrolled over relatively long periods of time and may never be performed [17]. Pragmatically, early initiation of dialysis should be implemented, since there are no data to show that it is harmful.

The real world and the indications for vascular access

The placement of vascular access should be considered when the GFR is <30ml/minute and created when the GFR is ≤20ml/minute with a view to starting dialysis when the GFR is <15ml/minute. However, implementing this is more difficult.

Perhaps the easiest problem to tackle is the patient (and sometimes the doctor) who is reluctant to start dialysis and undergo formation of arteriovenous access. Reluctance often stems from fear, not only of the unknown but also of the process itself and the disruption to patient and family life. Nearly all renal units now have predialysis or low clearance clinics, which are primarily run by nurses. These protocol-driven clinics have an important role and frequently overcome the barriers of fear and ignorance by involving counsellors, patient associations, other patients and their families. Close follow-up, based on simple protocols, ensures that many of the problems of renal failure such as hypertension, anaemia and bone disease are promptly treated. Plans for access creation can be organised and implemented through these clinics.

Inadequate resources for the creation of dialysis access and the provision of adequate haemodialysis facilities are more problematic. However, it is becoming increasingly recognised that access failure and access-associated problems are the major causes of hospital admission, morbidity and mortality in ESRF. In order to minimise hospitalisation, all renal units should have dedicated access surgeons and or radiologists. In North America, a new breed of nephrologist (the interventional nephrologist) is emerging with a special remit to create, maintain and monitor vascular access. Because of the lack of satellite-based haemodialysis facilities in the UK, peritoneal dialysis (either continuous ambulatory peritoneal dialysis [CAPD] or automated peritoneal dialysis [APD]) is often used as a short or medium-term solution for many patients. The realisation of this has resulted in a recent expansion in these facilities, which is likely to continue with the implementation of the Renal National Service Framework.

Conclusions

In the ideal world, the indications for the creation of vascular access are simple. A GFR of less than 30ml/minute should trigger a plan of action for the creation of vascular access. A GFR of less than 20ml/minute should result in the timely placement of vascular access. The real world is often different and this simple algorithm may be made more complex by patient choice and the availability of the appropriate resources for access surgery and haemodialysis.

Key Summary

◆ The simplest and most robust methods of measuring GFR are the plasma creatinine and formulae derived from the creatinine with the understanding that they overestimate true GFR.

◆ In an ideal world, vascular access should be planned and created well before it is needed and the patient has become significantly symptomatic from uraemia.

◆ In general, vascular access should be planned when the GFR is <30ml/minute, access should be created when the GFR is ≤20ml/minute and dialysis started when the GFR is <15ml/minute.

References

1. Melloni's Illustrated Medical Dictionary. 4th Edition. Parthenon Press, 2002.
2. The New Shorter Oxford English Dictionary. Oxford: Oxford University Press, 1993.
3. Cameron JS, Greger R. In: *Oxford Textbook of Clinical Nephrology*. 2nd Edition. Chapter 1.3: 39-69. Davidson AM, Cameron JS, Grunfield J-P, Kerr DNS, Ritz E, Winearls O, Eds. Oxford: Oxford University Press, 1998.
4. Stevens LA, Coresh J, Greene T, Levey AS. Assessing kidney function - measured and estimated glomerular filtration rate. *New Engl J Med* 2006; 354: 2473-83.
5. Shemesh O, Golbetz H, Kriss JP, Myers BD. Limitations of creatinine as a filtration marker in glomerulopathic patients. *Kidney Int* 1985; 28: 830-8.
6. Giovannetti S, Barsotti G. In defence of creatinine clearance. *Nephron* 1991; 59: 11-4.
7. Cockcroft DW, Gault MH. Prediction of creatinine clearance from serum creatinine. *Nephron* 1976; 16: 31-41.
8. Levey AS, Bosch JP, Breyer Lewis J, *et al.* A more accurate method to estimate glomerular filtration rate from serum creatinine: a new prediction equation. Modification of Diet in Renal Disease Study Group. *Ann Internal Med* 1999; 130: 461-70.

9.   Ritsch L, Blumberg A, Huber A. Rapid and accurate assessment of glomerular filtration rate in patients with renal transplants using serum cystatin C. *Nephrol Dial Transplant* 1999; 14: 1991-6.

10.   Deinum J, Derkx FHM. Cystatin for estimation of glomerular filtration rate. *Lancet* 2000; 356: 1624-5.

11.   Tattersall J, Geenwood R, Farrington K. Urea kinetics and when to start dialysis. *Am J Nephrol* 1995; 15: 283-9.

12.   NKF-K-DOQI Clinical Practice Guidelines for Haemodialysis Adequacy; Update 2000. *Am J Kidney Dis* 2001; 37: S7-S64.

13.   Mitch WE, Walser M, Buffington GA, Lemann J. A simple method of estimating the progression of chronic renal failure. *Lancet* 1976; 2: 1326-8.

14.   Shah BV, Levey AS. Spontaneous changes in the rate of decline in reciprocal serum creatinine; errors in predicting the progression of renal disease from extrapolation of the slope. *J Am Soc Nephrol* 1992; 11: 86-91.

15.   Rocco MV, Gassman JJ, Wang SR, Kaplan RM. Cross-sectional study of quality of life and symptoms in chronic renal disease patients: The Modification of Diet in Renal Disease Study. *Am J Kidney Dis* 1997; 29: 888-96.

16.   Churchill DN. An evidence-based approach to earlier initiation of dialysis. *Am J Kidney Dis* 1997; 30: 899-906.

17.   Traynor JP, Simpson K, Geddes CC, *et al.* Early initiation of dialysis fails to prolong survival in patients with endstage renal failure. *J Am Soc Nephrol* 2002; 13: 2125-32.

Chapter 3
Vascular access surgery: how much is needed?

Andrew J Williams MD FRCP

Consultant Nephrologist, Morriston Hospital, Swansea, UK

Introduction

The overwhelming majority of patients treated with renal replacement therapy for either acute or chronic established renal failure (ERF) receive haemodialysis at some stage and, as a result, require access to their circulation. The number of vascular surgical procedures needed is dependent on the incidence and prevalence of renal replacement therapy and on the type of vascular access used for haemodialysis.

Despite the potential benefits of renal transplantation for the majority of patients with chronic ERF, the shortage of kidneys limits its availability. The introduction in the late 1970s of Continuous Ambulatory Peritoneal Dialysis (CAPD) and other forms of chronic peritoneal dialysis has provided an alternative mode of dialysis treatment for those patients who have not received a successful renal transplant. However, with time, changes occur in the peritoneal membrane, which result in loss of effective dialysis so that relatively few patients are able to maintain adequate dialysis using the peritoneum for more than five years. As a result the haemodialysis population continues to rise.

The importance of vascular access to patients with ERF was well recognised by nephrologists practising in the 1970s, many of whom cared for patients who ultimately died as a result of failure to gain access to the circulation.

Since it was introduced in 1966, the Brescia-Cimino arteriovenous (AV) fistula has been the gold standard against which other forms of vascular access are compared. However, in most patients it takes several weeks for the fistula to mature sufficiently to allow reliable use and in some patients construction is difficult or precluded by the vascular anatomy. For these reasons alternative means of access to the circulation have been used in many patients.

The polytetrafluoroethylene (PTFE) graft was originally developed as an arterial conduit, but became widely used in the 1970s as a means of access for haemodialysis when placed between an upper limb artery and vein. The introduction of double-lumen catheters for central venous cannulation in the early 1980s enabled emergency treatment of patients for whom it would previously have been impossible. Although the availability of these techniques has enabled treatment of many patients who would previously not have been accepted onto renal replacement programs, there is concern that their widespread use for long-term dialysis is not beneficial for patients. Prosthetic arteriovenous grafts have inferior patency rates by comparison with AV fistulae and are associated with an increased need for corrective surgery. Central venous catheters are associated with a high rate of complications [1] that include infection, thrombosis and vessel stenosis. This was clearly demonstrated in one study [2] that showed that central venous catheters and arteriovenous grafts were respectively associated with approximately 50% and 26% increased mortality by comparison with AV fistulae in 616 incident haemodialysis patients for up to three years of follow-up.

In recognition of this, various bodies have assessed the benefits and disadvantages of the different modes of vascular access and produced recommendations for good practice.

Standards for vascular access

As a result of the excess morbidity and mortality associated with the use of grafts and venous catheters for vascular access in the US, the National Kidney Foundation included a vascular access section in their Dialysis Outcomes Quality Initiative (DOQI) [3]. Their recommendations are now widely quoted as the standard against which clinical practice regarding vascular access for haemodialysis should be guided. The advice given in the section "Clinical practice guidelines for vascular access" is:

◆ the order of preference for placement of AV fistulae in patients requiring chronic haemodialysis is:
  ● a wrist (radial-cephalic) primary AV fistula;
  ● an elbow (brachial-cephalic) primary AV fistula;
◆ if it is not possible to establish either of these types of fistula, access may be established using:
  ● an arteriovenous graft of synthetic material (e.g. PTFE); or
  ● a transposed brachial-basilic vein fistula;
◆ cuffed tunnelled central venous catheters should be discouraged as permanent vascular access.

More recently, similar guidelines have been adopted by other national bodies [4] and the UK Renal Association [5] recommends that:

◆ at least 67% of patients who had presented more than three months before starting haemodialysis should start dialysis with a usable native AV fistula;
◆ at least 80% of prevalent haemodialysis patients should be dialysed using a native AV fistula;
◆ no patient already requiring dialysis should wait more than four weeks for fistula construction including those who present late.

Current practice

Since the publication of the DOQI guidelines interest has centred on the extent to which they are deliverable. Up until recently national and international registries allowed analysis of the number of patients undergoing the different modes of renal replacement therapy, but generally did not provide sufficient detail on which to base an assessment of vascular access practice.

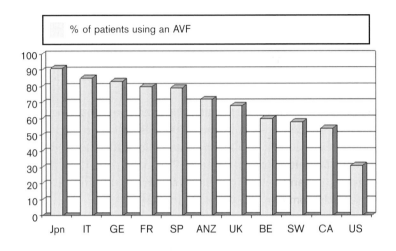

Figure 1 Autogenous AV fistula use in prevalent haemodialysis patients.

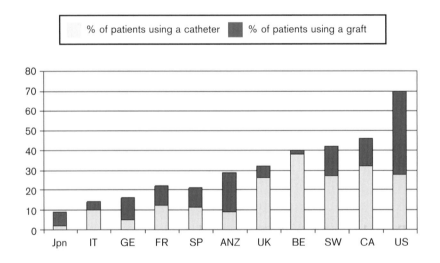

Figure 2 Central venous catheter and graft use in prevalent haemodialysis patients.

The Dialysis Outcomes and Practice Patterns Study (DOPPS) was designed to address some of the limitations of international registries and is a prospective, longitudinal study of haemodialysis practice and associated outcomes. The first phase of the study (DOPPS 1, 1996-2001) [6] collected data from France, Germany, Italy, Japan, Spain, the UK and the US. The second phase (DOPPS 11, 2002-2004) [7] included five additional countries (Australia, Belgium, Canada, New Zealand and Sweden) and emphasises the differences in practice that exist between North America and elsewhere (Figure 1), with much greater use of AV fistulae in the latter even when adjusted for case mix. The percentage of prevalent haemodialysis patients who receive dialysis with a graft or catheter also differs markedly from one country to another (Figure 2) [8].

Even within individual countries practice can differ markedly from one centre to another. In the UK, 69% of prevalent haemodialysis patients in 2005 were dialysed using either an AV fistula (65.6%) or a graft (4.3%), but the range from one unit to another was large (44-94%) [9].

As well as geographic factors reported in the DOPPS study there are several demographic and clinical factors that have been associated with differences in the use of AV fistulae for haemodialysis. A lower prevalence of fistulae is found in females than in males, in blacks than in whites and in the old than in the young. Clinical factors associated with a lower prevalence of fistulae include the presence of peripheral vascular disease and obesity.

The failure of the US to meet the DOQI guidelines highlights the enormous challenge that vascular access presents on a worldwide basis [10].

Prevalence of end-stage renal disease

Based on information [11] obtained from 122 countries with a combined population of 6.4 billion (92% of the world population), it has been estimated that at the end of 2004 there were 1,783,000 patients worldwide undergoing renal replacement therapy for established renal

Table 1 Prevalence of treated established renal failure in 24 different countries in 2004 [11].

Country	Grafts (pmp)	HD (pmp)	PD (pmp)	Total ERF (pmp)
Phillipines	-	44	8	52
Russia	23	75	6	102
Thailand	25	203	15	243
Turkey	47	340	46	433
Iceland	253	140	86	479
Malaysia	62	417	43	522
Hungary	211	384	27	622
Finland	410	218	57	685
Netherlands	379	242	83	704
Australia	312	307	88	707
Norway	513	162	33	708
New Zealand	301	250	186	737
Denmark	303	351	115	769
Sweden	425	291	84	800
Chile	156	644	41	841
Korea	183	517	154	854
Austria	417	408	33	858
Luxembourg	457	454	-	911
Greece	168	684	70	922
Germany	258	702	38	998
Italy	263	668	91	1022
USA	464	1014	85	1563
Taiwan	-	1575	131	1706
Japan	-	1788	69	1857

HD=Haemodialysis
PD=Peritoneal dialysis
ERF=Established renal failure

failure. Of these, 412,000 had a functioning renal transplant, 1,222,000 were undergoing haemodialysis and 149,000 were treated with peritoneal dialysis. These numbers are 20% higher than those reported in the equivalent survey for the year 2001. The resulting average global prevalence of treated ERF (i.e. total number of patients per million population [pmp] with renal transplants or receiving dialysis for chronic renal failure) was 280 patients pmp, of whom 215 patients pmp were receiving dialysis.

There is enormous disparity (Table 1) between the situation in several developing countries in which the prevalence is <10 pmp and the situation in the US, Taiwan and Japan where the prevalence is 1,563 patients pmp, 1,706 patients pmp and 1,857 patients pmp, respectively [12]. At the end of 2004, 52% of the global dialysis population was treated in just four countries (USA, Japan, Brazil and Germany), which together accounted for only 11% of the world population.

The prevalence of renal replacement therapy for ERF continues to rise in all countries that are able to run renal replacement programs. The total dialysis population worldwide rose by 6% during 2004, although the rate of increase is greater (approximately 10%) in those countries with a relatively low prevalence of treated ERF.

In the UK, the estimated (The UK Renal Registry; Eighth Annual Report; December 2005) prevalence of renal replacement therapy in December 2004 was 638 patients pmp. The prevalence of patients receiving dialysis varied from 172 to 625 pmp in different parts of the country, with 76% undergoing haemodialysis in December 2004.

Factors influencing the prevalence of treated ERF

The variation in prevalence of renal replacement therapy between different countries in part reflects the distribution of wealth and the ability of the countries to provide the economic support for a treatment program. Nevertheless, amongst economically well developed countries such as those in the European Union, there is a spectrum of prevalence suggesting that these discrepancies may truly reflect differences in the incidence of

ERF rather than the ability of countries to support a treatment program from an economic perspective.

The incidence of ERF in a given population is dependent on various factors, which include the age distribution, sex, ethnicity and degree of deprivation. In the UK, the incidence of renal replacement therapy rises from about 50 new patients pmp in the 35-39 year age group to 150 in the 55-59 year age group and 450 in the 75-79 year age group. There is an excess of males in the over 40s which rises with increasing age thereafter. The non-Caucasian population has a significantly higher (approximately four-fold) incidence of ERF in the UK than the Caucasian population. Similarly, in the US, African Americans have an incidence of ERF which is at least four times greater than that of the white population. This discrepancy in part reflects a higher prevalence of diabetes and hypertension in the Indo-Asian and Afro-Caribbean populations. These factors have a major impact on the prevalence of ERF and hence requirements for renal replacement therapy in areas with either an elderly population or high proportion of non-Caucasians.

As well as being directly related to the incidence of ERF the prevalence of renal replacement therapy is influenced by patient survival once treatment is started. In the past there have been clearly demonstrated differences in survival between haemodialysed patients in the US and in Europe. These may have been due in part to differences in treatment protocols with a tendency towards a reduction in the dose of dialysis delivered in the US, which may have prejudiced survival. Other possible explanations include the greater use of AV fistulae for dialysis in European dialysis centres [2, 13].

Another factor that has a significant impact on the prevalence of renal replacement therapy is the age of onset of renal disease. In non-Caucasians renal disease generally occurs at a younger age than in Caucasians. This will tend to increase the prevalence of treated ERF in developing countries if treatment is no longer rationed by economic consideration.

Improvements in treatment will continue to increase the number of patients treated for ERF and it has been predicted that by 2010 there will be about 2.0 million patients worldwide undergoing chronic dialysis.

Surgical workload implications of vascular access

It is generally accepted that AV fistulae should be used for vascular access whenever possible and the value of a high quality vascular and peritoneal access service to a renal unit is immense. Surgical expertise and enthusiasm is paramount to its success but without adequate resource, including beds and operating theatre time, enthusiasm alone cannot be expected to cope with the increasing workload.

Recent UK guidelines have advised that there should be dedicated theatre sessions for access surgery sufficient to provide one session per week for every 120 patients on dialysis. With this level of access surgery provision it is hoped that no patient on dialysis, including those who present late, should wait for more than four weeks for AV fistula construction.

The relationship between vascular access workload and the number of new dialysis patients per year alters as the size (i.e. prevalence of treated ERF) of the renal replacement program increases. Hence, the factors that influence the workload for the surgeon include:

◆ number of new dialysis patients (incidence of ERF) per year and the proportion of them undergoing haemo- or peritoneal dialysis;
◆ total number (prevalence) of dialysis patients. Of these a proportion will require:
  ● revision / re-do of vascular access;
  ● replacement of peritoneal access;
  ● conversion from peritoneal dialysis to haemodialysis and vice versa;
◆ number of patients with a renal transplant. In a proportion of these (approximately 3% of the total transplant population per annum) the transplant will fail and the patient may require vascular or peritoneal access in order to be re-established on dialysis.

Given the complex relationship between these different components of a renal replacement program, it is not possible to accurately predict the number of procedures that are needed on an annual basis. As well as the influence that the incidence and prevalence of the different modes of treatment have on operative workload, local surgical and radiological practice can have a significant impact. For example, a surgeon who puts great emphasis on using distal vessels whenever possible is likely to have a higher 're-do' rate than a surgeon who is less enthusiastic about preserving vessels.

However, some indication can be gained from previous experience and be adapted to local circumstance. During a 13-year period (1989-2002) in a UK renal unit (catchment population 750,000), where less than 10% of haemodialysed patients were using central venous catheters at any one time, 1237 vascular access procedures (771 patients) and 897 peritoneal dialysis procedures (insertion or removal) were performed by a single surgeon. The number of new patients taken onto the program rose steadily from 60 per annum in 1989 to 114 in 2002. The number of dialysed patients rose from 102 (haemodialysis: 69; peritoneal dialysis: 33) to 279 (haemodialysis: 184; peritoneal dialysis: 95) in 2002. The number of patients with functioning transplants rose from 105 in 1989 to 240 in 2002.

Of the vascular procedures, 448 (420 primary) were snuffbox AV fistulae, 420 (232 primary) were radiocephalic AV fistulae, 272 (98 primary) were brachial AV fistulae and 16 (six primary) were ulnar AV fistulae. Eighteen vein loops were performed and four patients underwent basilic vein transposition. Thirty-two PTFE grafts (28 forearm; three upper arm; one thigh) were inserted and 27 other procedures (e.g. exploration without AVF; revisions; operations for steal) were undertaken. During this time the number of procedures (vascular plus peritoneal access) required on an annual basis was approximately:

(Incidence + Prevalence of Dialysed Patients) / 2

Thus, for 2002, the predicted number of procedures required would be (114 + 279)/2 = 197. Assuming an average of three procedures can be performed on a dedicated access operating list, 66 operating sessions would be required per year.

Extrapolating this to UK incidence (103 pmp) and prevalence (351 pmp) rates for 2004, it would suggest the need for 227 procedures (76 operating sessions) per annum pmp to maintain the status quo. However, it is important to recognise that incidence and, more especially, prevalence of renal replacement therapy, is rising and also that in many units there are a large number of patients dialysing with intravenous catheters at present who would add to the workload if they were to have AV fistulae constructed.

In this regard it is of note that the DOPPS investigators showed in both the US and Europe that AV fistulae lasted longer than grafts, when either had been used as the patients' initial mode of vascular access. Furthermore, it was found that both survived longer if used as the patients' first mode of vascular access than when used after dialysis had been started using a catheter.

Finally, vascular surgical workload can be significantly reduced if other health professionals ensure that veins are preserved whenever possible and that AV fistulae and grafts are given close observation and meticulous care.

Conclusions

There is no doubt that the number of patients treated with dialysis worldwide is going to continue to increase during the foreseeable future and the vast majority of these patients will require vascular access for haemodialysis. As the prevalence of treated ERF rises, the already considerable workload for the surgeons who work alongside nephrologists will continue to rise and will present a major challenge for those planning renal replacement programs for the future.

Key Summary

◆ Arteriovenous fistulae are the preferred mode of vascular access for patients undergoing long-term haemodialysis and should be used in at least 80% of prevalent patients.

◆ The DOPP Study has shown serious deficiencies in the UK and US, with respect to the "standards for vascular access" published by the UK Renal Association and the National Kidney Foundation in their Dialysis Outcomes Quality Initiative.

◆ The total dialysis population rises by 6% per annum worldwide and at the end of 2004 there were more than 1.2 million patients being treated with haemodialysis. The rate of increase is greatest in those countries with a relatively low prevalence of treated ERF and it is predicted that by 2010 there will be more than two million patients treated with dialysis.

References

1. Dhingra RK, Young EW, Hulbert-Shearon TE, *et al.* Type of vascular access and mortality in US hemodialysis patients. *Kidney Int* 2001; 60: 1443-51.
2. Astor BC, Eustace JA, Powe NR, *et al.* Type of vascular access and survival among incident hemodialysis patients: The Choices for Healthy Outcomes in Caring for ESRD (CHOICE) Study. *J Am Soc Nephrol* 2005; 16: 1449-55.
3. NKF-K/DOQI Clinical Practice Guidelines for Vascular Access: Update 2000. *Am J Kidney Dis* 2001; 37: S137-S181.
4. Jindal K, Chan CT, Deziel C, *et al.* Haemodialysis clinical practice guidelines for the Canadian Society of Nephrology. Vascular Access. *J Am Soc Nephrol* 2006; 17: S16-S23.
5. Treatment of adults and children with renal failure. Standards and audit measures. 3rd Edition. The Renal Association, 2002.

6.   Pisoni RL, Young EW, Dykstra DM, *et al.* Vascular access use in Europe and the United States. Results from the DOPPS. *Kidney Int* 2002; 61: 305-16.

7.   Port FK, Pisoni RL, Bommer J, *et al.* Improving outcomes for dialysis patients in the international Dialysis Outcomes and Practice Patterns Study. *Clin J Am Soc Nephrol* 2006; 1: 246-55.

8.   Roy-Chaudhury P, Sukhatme VP, Cheung AK. Hemodialysis vascular access dysfunction: a cellular and molecular viewpoint. *J Am Soc Nephrol* 2006; 17: 1112-27.

9.   The UK Renal Registry. The Eighth Annual Report. December 2005. The National Dialysis Access Survey - preliminary results.

10.   Allon M, Robbin ML. Increasing arteriovenous fistulas in hemodialysis patients: problems and solutions. *Kidney Int* 2002; 62: 1109-24.

11.   Grassmann A, Gioberge S, Moeller S, Brown G. ESRD patients in 2004: global overview of patient numbers, treatment modalities and associated trends. *Nephrol Dial Transplant* 2005; 20: 2587-93.

12.   United States Renal Data System. Annual Data Report, 2006: Chapter 12.

13.   Ishani A, Collins AJ, Herzog CA, Foley RN. Septicaemia, access and cardiovascular disease in dialysis patients: the USRDS Wave 2 study. *Kidney Int* 2005; 68: 311-8.

Chapter 4
Temporary vascular access

Peter Choi MA MB PhD MRCP, *Consultant Nephrologist*
Andrew H Frankel Bsc MB BS MD FRCP, *Consultant Nephrologist*
West London Renal and Transplant Centre, Hammersmith Hospital, London, UK

Introduction

A major goal in the management of haemodialysis patients is to establish and maintain definitive long-term vascular access, in the form of autogenous arteriovenous (AV) fistulae or prosthetic AV grafts. However, there are situations when vascular access is required for a defined or limited period. These may include:

◆ acute renal failure - where early recovery is anticipated;
◆ the initial management of unheralded chronic renal failure;
◆ a bridging modality between different forms of renal replacement therapy;
◆ a bridging modality while permanent access is being planned, revised or is maturing;
◆ non-dialysis nephrological indications (plasma exchange).

In the early years of the renal replacement program, Scribner AV shunts were widely employed for immediate vascular access in renal patients. However, their use has declined significantly over the last two decades and there has been a loss in the expertise available to perform and maintain these shunts. Haemodialysis catheters have emerged as the major means of achieving quick and efficient access to the vascular compartment. Although the change to haemodialysis catheters has been seen as a positive development, they are not without risk of complications. Haemodialysis catheters can be inserted directly into a major vein (non-tunnelled) or, alternatively, they can be tunnelled subcutaneously.

Currently, non-tunnelled catheters are the predominant access solution used where urgent or temporary access to the circulation is required. However, there is likely to be wider use of tunnelled haemodialysis catheters for these situations in the future, particularly as units enlarge and develop multidisciplinary teams between physicians, surgeons and radiologists.

The use of non-tunnelled, as opposed to tunnelled haemodialysis catheters varies from unit to unit. Data from the 8th UK Renal Registry Report [1] indicates that a significant number of units rely on non-tunnelled haemodialysis catheters when establishing patients on treatment, and 36% of patients commencing treatment in 2005 started with a non-tunnelled catheter (Table 1). A review of vascular access practice across the UK [2] indicates that while this situation is often because of late referral, it is also due to organisational issues within renal units including problems relating to referral and access to surgical lists. While improvements in referral, planning and organisation will result in a reduction in the number of patients who require non-tunnelled lines, this situation is likely to continue. Therefore, individual units should have a policy for the management of emergency and temporary vascular access, and haemodialysis catheters in particular, that produces the lowest morbidity. In order to adequately define such a policy, it is important to understand the relative advantages and disadvantages of tunnelled and non-tunnelled haemodialysis catheters when used for temporary access.

Table 1 Type of access at first treatment for end-stage renal failure in UK renal units during April 2005 [1].

Access type	Number of patients	% of patients
AVF	104	30
Graft	6	2
Non-tunnelled catheter	126	36
Tunnelled catheter	115	33

Catheter design

The design of non-tunnelled haemodialysis catheters has evolved over time from single-lumen catheters, which were introduced into a separate artery and vein, to the subsequent development of dual-lumen haemodialysis catheters. This has been such a success that for many years the standard design has remained unmodified.

Dual-lumen catheters have two coaxial lumens positioned within a single catheter. The arterial port is generally 2-3cm proximal to the venous port. There are differences in design between different catheters, including differences in size, extension ports, antibiotic coating, etc. These design differences only become clinically significant in patients who require prolonged use of temporary access.

Most modern dual-lumen non-tunnelled haemodialysis catheters are formed from polyurethane, which is stiff at room temperature, but which softens at body temperature, reducing the risk of vascular damage. Soft silicone is also employed for the construction of tunnelled and non-tunnelled haemodialysis catheters. While stiff polyurethane catheters can be inserted via a guidewire using the Seldinger technique, softer silicone catheters require insertion through a peel-away sheath.

Non-tunnelled haemodialysis catheters are available in a variety of lengths, from 12-24cm. It is important to assess the length of the catheter required for individual patients. This is dependent on the patient's size, and the site of insertion of the catheter. Generally, longer catheters are required for insertion via the left internal jugular and femoral routes, in order to ensure that the catheter tip lies in the correct position (see below).

Catheter diameter varies between 11-14 French (Fr.). Older designs utilised smaller lumens (11-12 Fr.), which placed significant limitations on the maximal blood flow achieved, since Poiseuille's equation indicates that an increase in intraluminal radius results in an exponential increase in blood flow. In order to achieve the targets for dialysis adequacy currently recommended by UK and US national guidelines, blood flows on dialysis >350ml per minute are required. This is of particular importance in patients who are being maintained on chronic haemodialysis, where larger-bore

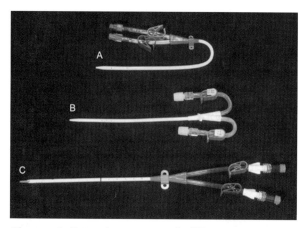

Figure 1 Extension ports of different temporary haemodialysis catheters illustrating: a) a precurved dialysis catheter with straight extensions suitable for the internal jugular route; b) precurved extensions on a straight catheter suitable for internal jugular route; c) a standard catheter with straight extensions suitable for femoral or subclavian route.

catheters have considerable advantages. Catheter diameter is relatively less important in patients who are dialysed for acute renal failure, or where the indication for cannulation is strictly temporary.

An important difference in design of non-tunnelled catheters relates to external extensions, which may be curved or straight (Figure 1). These affect patient comfort and the risk of infection, so that when used via the internal jugular route, the catheter hubs are kept away from the hairline.

Unlike non-tunnelled catheters there are fundamentally different types of tunnelled catheter on the market. The original generation of tunnelled haemodialysis catheters were dual-lumen tunnel haemodialysis catheters, which were silicone-based. Over the years adaptations were made to catheter design in order to achieve increasing flow rates. The original dual-lumen catheters have been redesigned and have evolved into split catheters, of which the Tesio catheter is the ultimate version, being entirely split in two catheters (Figure 2).

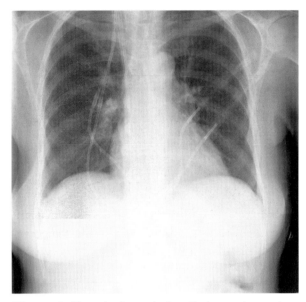

Figure 2 The design of the Tesio catheter has evolved back to utilising two separate catheters each inserted into the vein and tunnelled subcutaneously.

Tunnelled catheters can all be used for both short and long-term haemodialysis and, whereas previously, temporary dialysis was primarily undertaken using non-tunnelled catheters, given the reduced infection rate, tunnelled catheters have an equal role to play in the management of temporary haemodialysis.

Insertion

Haemodialysis catheters should be easily inserted into large veins with the minimum of short and long-term complications. Both the site and technique of insertion may influence catheter performance and the incidence of complications.

Technically, the internal jugular and femoral veins represent the easiest veins to access blindly and are the safest routes for insertion. The right internal jugular vein has been considered the prime route for haemodialysis catheters and is easier to access compared to the left internal jugular route. This is probably due to the fact that cannulation of the left internal jugular vein requires navigation of two right-hand turns, with the risk of placement of the catheter tip into the azygos vein (Figure 3). This may explain why left internal jugular catheters are associated with a significantly greater incidence of poor function and four times the need for replacement compared to the right.

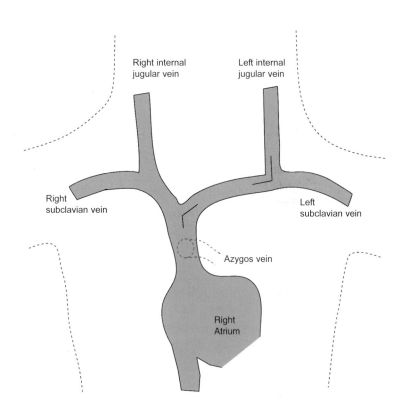

Figure 3 Anatomical representation of the route taken by a catheter inserted into the left internal jugular vein, illustrating the double right angle route required.

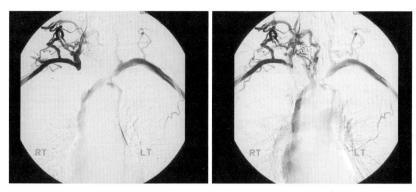

Figure 4 Central venous occlusion in a patient who had previously required temporary dialysis via a subclavian non-tunnelled haemodialysis catheter for the acute commencement of renal replacement therapy. (Both images were taken at different time points during the same study, highlighting the collateral vessels).

The subclavian route used to be considered the primary route for temporary haemodialysis access. However, there is a considerably greater risk of acute vessel damage during insertion and it has become apparent that there is a significant medium-term risk of developing subclavian venous stenosis (Figure 4). Studies dating back to the late 1980s demonstrated that angiograms, performed two to three weeks after insertion of subclavian haemodialysis catheters, revealed the presence of subclavian stenosis or obstruction in 40-50% of cases. Schillinger et al [3] studied patients with subclavian temporary haemodialysis catheters and found that there was a 42% subclavian stenosis rate compared to 10% for internal jugular lines. Catheters in this study were *in situ* for only 31 days and patients had undergone a mean of only 13 haemodialysis sessions. Subclavian stenosis has been postulated to arise from endothelial trauma, caused by the rhythmic rubbing of the line against the vein wall during the haemodialysis blood pump cycle. Once present, subclavian stenosis has a significant impact on the long-term ability to form permanent vascular access in the ipsilateral arm. The incidence of stenosis or obstruction associated with left internal jugular haemodialysis catheters, as compared to right internal jugular catheters, is unknown. Furthermore, there are no data to indicate whether the newer generation of split-line tunnelled haemodialysis catheters results in equivalent damage.

A number of other routes for access may be used in extremis. These include direct IVC cannulation via the translumbar or transhepatic approach and external jugular vein cannulation. Experience in the translumbar approach is increasing, but is not a primary route for short-term access to the circulation.

The Seldinger technique has been considered to be a routine bedside procedure and is usually carried out in a blind fashion, using anatomical landmarks to identify the probable route of the veins. The perception that this is a safe procedure is not confirmed by data relating to short-term complications (Table 2). However, ultrasound visualisation of the vein can greatly reduce the incidence of these complications. This is particularly helpful for patients, such as those on long-term haemodialysis, whose veins have been recurrently cannulated, and may have become tortuous or thrombosed. In addition, up to 25% of patients have anomalous internal jugular vein anatomy and blind cannulation of these individuals carries a greater risk. Real time ultrasound visualisation considerably reduces the risk of complications and improves patient comfort (Figure 5). In a meta-

Table 2 The incidence of recognised complications following catheter insertion into a major vein.

Complication	Incidence
Arterial puncture	0 - 12%
Pneumothorax	1 - 3%
Haemothorax	0.6%
Air embolism	<1%
Major bleed	<1%
Others Nerve palsy etc.	<1%

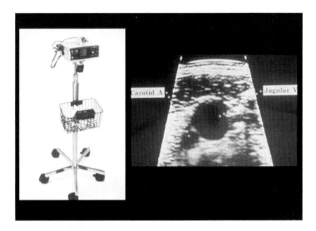

Figure 5 The SITE RITE 3[TM]* is one of the ultrasound devices available, which allows real time visualisation of the internal jugular vein. The images obtained allow clear definition of the internal jugular vein and its relationship to the carotid artery.

*SITE RITE 3 (Dymax Corporation, a subsidiary of Bard Access Systems).

analysis of catheter insertion procedures, Randolph et al[4] concluded that the use of ultrasound guidance was associated with a significantly reduced incidence of catheter insertion complications (relative risk 0.22) and placement failures (relative risk 0.32). The UK National Institute for Clinical Excellence (NICE-September 2002) and the US DOQI Committee have both recommended that two-dimensional ultrasound guidance is the preferred method for the insertion of central venous catheters into the internal jugular vein.

It is important to ensure that the catheter has been inserted appropriately so that its tip lies in a position that will deliver adequate blood flow. For internal jugular and subclavian routes this should be at the junction of the SVC and the right atrium. Given that non-tunnelled haemodialysis catheters formed from polyurethane are generally stiff at insertion, one should not aim to insert them into the right atrium, as the risk of right atrial wall damage is significant. In contrast, the softer, silicone-based permanent lines may be safely inserted into the right atrium. For a femoral approach, it is important to aim to position the tip of the catheter into the IVC. Generally, 20-24cm lines are required to avoid excessive recirculation. The position of the catheter tip should be checked either by fluoroscopy at the time of insertion or by radiology following insertion.

The major complication of haemodialysis catheters relates to their associated incidence of infection. There is a considerable amount of data that confirms the increased incidence of infection in patients with haemodialysis catheters, as compared to AV fistulae. When considering the management of temporary haemodialysis, the fact that tunnelled lines carry a significantly lower rate of infection than non-tunnelled lines should be paramount [5].

In selecting the most appropriate approach to the management of a patient requiring temporary or urgent haemodialysis (in whom no permanent access is *in situ*), one should consider the likely duration of treatment. If this is less than one week and the patient is hospitalised, the use of a femoral catheter could be considered. However, if treatment is likely to continue for longer, a non-tunnelled femoral catheter, followed by early insertion of a tunnelled internal jugular catheter is probably the optimum practice. Indeed if the unit has established appropriate systems in place, tunnelled lines may be used directly.

Catheter function

There are very little data to advise clinicians on which particular catheter to use. Tunnelled haemodialysis catheters, such as the Bard Optiflow, have been shown to perform better in comparison with first generation catheters such as the Hickman, with a reduced failure rate [6]. However, a variety of other studies have been undertaken which compared Optiflow with the Ash-split and the Tesio. These have shown little significant difference in function, although Richard *et al* concluded that the Ash-split and Tesio had a lower infection rate than the Optiflow and the Ash-split had the best longevity, but none of these catheters had any difference in flow rates [7]. Theoretically, Tesio and other split catheters are likely to have a reduced rate of thrombosis and therefore may have a lower incidence of central vein stenosis with wall trauma. However, there are little data available to confirm this theoretical advantage.

While catheter function is an extremely important pre-requisite when planning for long-term haemodialysis, high catheter flow rates are not necessarily vital for temporary haemodialysis for short periods of time. However, poor catheter function has significant implications for patient quality of life and nursing practice, as frequent machine alarms and the resulting interruption to haemodialysis and interventions require significant extensions of dialysis time and significant hands-on use of nursing time. This causes inconvenience for patients, cost to units and associated morbidity.

In order to understand why a catheter may be poorly performing, a full clinical assessment is required to diagnose the cause of dysfunction. Generally, catheter dysfunction can be classified into early or late dysfunction, each of which have different implications for management.

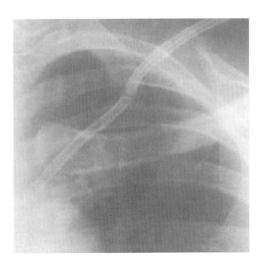

Early catheter dysfunction is that which never achieves a flow rate of greater than 300ml per minute. This is almost always due to unsatisfactory positioning, for instance with the catheter being placed in the azygos vein, and this should not occur if the catheter has been placed under fluoroscopic control. Kinking does, however, occur and may not be immediately picked up at insertion (Figure 6). Another factor that can affect immediate function is catheter

Figure 6 Catheter flow will usually be poor from the time of the first treatment (early catheter dysfunction) if there is kinking of the catheter.

retraction. This occurs most usually in obese patients, particularly women with tunnelled catheters. In this situation, when the patient lies prone the catheter may be in an excellent position. However, as the patient stands up, the soft tissues pull the catheter and cause retraction, such that the catheter tip may no longer lie in an ideal position. This should be taken into account when placing catheters in large patients with pendulous breast tissue.

Catheters that initially perform well, but whose function deteriorates are classified as suffering late dysfunction and this is usually due to some form of thrombosis. The thrombosis may be intrinsic to the catheter and may be luminal, although this should not occur if the catheter/heparinsation regime is properly adhered to. Thrombosis around the tip can also lead to the formation of a fibrin sheath which encases the catheter. There is some theoretical advantage to Tesio and split catheters, which may be less likely to suffer from this complication, given that they have two separate catheters, which move apart during the course of the haemodialysis cycle. Extrinsic thrombosis, in which the vein in which the catheter sits has suffered a thrombosis, is usually associated with clinical features (fever, venous congestion, arm swelling, etc), compared to the asymptomatic development of intrinsic thrombosis.

In assessing a patient with diminishing catheter flow, it is vital to review initially the patient's fluid status, as volume depletion can cause poor catheter flow. The catheter position should also be checked and the patient should be reviewed for signs of central vein stenosis or infection. Initial management of a catheter that is believed to have suffered from thrombosis is to undertake a saline flush, which is often a temporary and incomplete measure. Switching of the lines is another temporary solution, which may result in an improvement in flow at the price of an increase in recirculation. This will tend to be less important in patients undergoing temporary haemodialysis than for long-term haemodialysis. The use of lytic or anti-thrombotic therapy can be used for tunnelled catheters. However, it is inappropriate treatment for patients with non-tunnelled catheters in whom the treatment should be to replace non-tunnelled catheters at the earliest opportunity.

For lytic therapy, both tissue plasminogen activator and urokinase have a very high success rate. They are used intraluminally or in a systemic fashion. However, rethrombosis often occurs. If a patient needs more than three treatments within a month, the tunnelled catheter should be replaced, as long-term viability is less likely [8].

Radiological support also has a role to play in the management of temporary catheter dysfunction. Radiological intervention can be used to reposition a catheter and also with the removal or stripping of any fibrin sheaf.

As discussed above, the goals of catheter function for temporary haemodialysis catheters may differ subtly from those required for long-term chronic haemodialysis. In the latter situation, haemodialysis adequacy is paramount, thus necessitating flow rates consistently >350ml per minute. In contrast, achieving adequacy targets in acute settings may not be so vital, although this should not dilute efforts to achieve optimal catheter function.

Conclusions

Temporary haemodialysis catheters are a necessary evil in the management of patients with renal disease, both acute and chronic. Their use should be minimised by the establishment of an adequate vascular access program and by early referral of patients with renal failure. Ideally, non-tunnelled haemodialysis catheters should not be used for longer than one week, and patients can be maintained on short-term femoral lines prior to insertion of tunnelled dialysis catheters. It is important that each dialysis unit has appropriate protocols defining insertion technique and the care and maintenance of the non-tunnelled haemodialysis catheter sites. Attention to detail in this area can have significant impact on both short and long-term morbidity in patients requiring renal replacement therapy.

Key Summary

◆ The use of non-tunnelled haemodialysis catheters should be minimised by early referral, a comprehensive and well managed vascular access program and by the ability to insert tunnelled catheters on a daily basis.

◆ Ideally, non-tunnelled catheters should not be used for more than one week.

◆ Catheter insertion should be planned to ensure that the correct catheter (tunnelled or non-tunnelled) is inserted into the most appropriate vein, by an experienced operator.

◆ Flow rates for tunnelled catheters should exceed 350ml/minute.

◆ The assessment of poor catheter function should be systematic and aim to identify the underlying cause.

References

1. UK Renal Registry Report, 2005. UK Renal Registry, Bristol, UK.
2. The National Dialysis Access Survey - Preliminary Results. Chapter 6. UK Renal Registry Report 2005. UK Renal Registry, Bristol, UK.
3. Schillinger F, Schillinger D, Montagnac R, Milcent T. Post-catheterisation vein stenosis in haemodialysis: comparative angiographic study of 50 subclavian and 50 internal jugular accesses. *Nephrol Dial Transplant* 1991; 6: 722-4.
4. Randolph AG, Cook DJ, Gonzales CA, Pribble CG. Ultrasound guidance for placement of central venous catheters: a meta-analysis of the literature. *Crit Care Med* 1996; 24: 2053-8.
5. Tokars JI, Miller ER, Stein G. New national surveillance system for haemodialysis-associated infections: initial results. *AJIC* 2002; 30: 288-95.
6. Rocklin MA, Dwight CA, Callen LJ, *et al*. Comparison of cuffed tunnelled haemodialysis catheter survival. *Am J Kidney Dis* 2001; 37(3): 557-63.
7. Richard HM, Hastings GS, Boyd-Kranis RL, *et al*. A randomised, prospective evaluation of the Tesio, Ash-split and Opti-flow haemodialysis catheters. *J Vasc Interv Radiol* 2001; 12(4): 431-5.
8. Little MA, Walshe JJ. A longitudinal study of the repeated use of alteplase as therapy for tunnelled haemodialysis catheter dysfunction. *Am J Kidney Dis* 2001; 39: 86-91.

Chapter 5

Radiological assessment prior to surgery

Peter WG Brown BSc FRCS FRCR

Consultant Radiologist, Sheffield Teaching Hospitals NHS Trust, Sheffield, UK

Introduction

In many centres patients presenting for primary access proceed directly to arteriovenous (AV) fistula formation after careful physical examination. If there is a satisfactory radial pulse and suitable forearm veins there is a good chance of success. Clinical guidelines provided by NKF-DOQI in 1997 state that imaging is only necessary in certain patients: venography is indicated where there is a suspicion of central vein stenosis or trauma, and in patients with multiple previous access attempts [1]. Ultrasound or MRI is suggested in certain complex cases or in pre-dialysis patients with minimal residual renal function where there is a risk of iodinated contrast causing acute renal failure. Rarely, angiography or arterial duplex are indicated when arterial pulses are diminished.

Despite these guidelines up to one third of access procedures will either thrombose or fail to mature sufficiently for dialysis. More widespread pre-operative imaging could reduce the rate of primary fistula failure and reduce unnecessary surgery. Traditional contrast venography was the gold standard for many years but its generalised use is limited by its relative invasiveness, risk of allergic reaction, contrast nephropathy and cost. More recently, there is evidence that pre-operative duplex ultrasound can not only increase the utilisation of native AV fistulae for dialysis access, but also allows optimal selection of AV fistula sites. Ultrasound is being increasingly utilised, as it is readily available and cheap but has a major limitation of being unable to assess central vein patency. Thus, contrast venography may still be needed if a central venous stenosis or occlusion is suspected. In those patients in whom iodinated contrast is contraindicated, magnetic resonance venography (MRV) and carbon dioxide venography have recently become available as alternatives. MRV can also give excellent anatomical detail of peripheral arm veins, although its relative lack of availability and high cost will probably prevent its widespread introduction.

Duplex ultrasound scanning

Technique

A high frequency linear phased array probe should be used with the arm dependent. Arterial and venous studies can be performed at the same time.

Venous study

The arm is scanned proximal to distal, with and without a tourniquet. Veins should be thin walled, vary in size with respiration, collapse completely on compression with the transducer, and augment with distal compression. Vessel depth, internal diameter with and without the tourniquet, continuity with the deep system, and the presence of any stenosis or thrombosis are assessed (Figure 1). Veins should dilate by

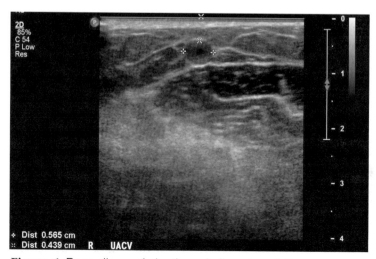

Figure 1 Recordings of depth and diameter of the upper arm cephalic vein (transverse section).

approximately 50% with a tourniquet. There should be respiratory variation in the subclavian vein and, if indicated, the venous flow rate can be recorded during unforced inspiration. Recordings of depth and diameter (with and without a tourniquet) should be recorded on a chart, which can be taken with the patient to theatre.

Arterial study

The arm is again scanned proximal to distal. Internal diameters are recorded at different levels, as well as calcification and abnormal arterial wall thickening, and noted on a chart. The arterial waveform should also be evaluated both proximally and distally and, in particular, at the site of the proposed AV fistula. Peak systolic velocities should be recorded. The normal waveform should be a triphasic, high resistance flow with no evidence of damping which could indicate a proximal stenosis.

Following AV fistula construction blood flow through the feeding artery is increased and the peripheral resistance is decreased because of diversion to the low resistance venous circulation. The Doppler waveform is changed from a triphasic high resistance waveform to a biphasic low resistance waveform with increased diastolic flow. Reactive hyperaemia

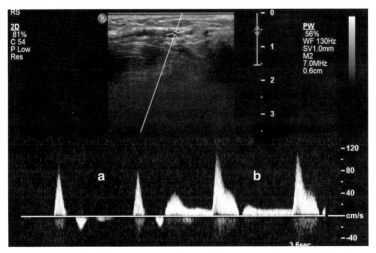

Figure 2 a) Radial artery waveform during clenched fist and b) on release, showing a hyperaemic response.

(RH) simulates the decreased vascular resistance after AV fistula construction and the Doppler waveform during RH can be used as a test for the ability of an artery to sustain the increased flow (Figure 2). RH can be induced by opening a fist after clenching for two minutes. The change in the waveform can be recorded by measuring the resistive index (RI), as well as changes in peak systolic and end diastolic velocity.

Criteria for successful AV fistula construction

Arterial diameter

The normal diameter of the radial artery is 2-3.5mm. A luminal diameter of less than 1.6mm [2] or 1.5mm [3] has been found to be associated with early fistula failure. Pre-operative radial artery diameters have been found to be smaller among patients with failed forearm fistulae compared with successful fistulae (1.9mm versus 2.8mm) [4]. A minimum diameter of 2mm is now usually advised [5]. Above this minimal diameter there seems to be no correlation between arterial diameter and fistula success.

Arterial flow and velocity

Adequate arterial inflow is crucial to the successful maturation of forearm fistulae but accurate pre-operative flow rates are difficult to measure due to the small diameter of the radial artery. Peak systolic velocity (PSV) of the proposed inflow artery is easier to measure and has also been evaluated as a predictor of a successful AV fistula. A PSV of at least 50cm/sec was found to be necessary for fistula success in one study [6]. In another study, in which arteries measuring <2mm in diameter were excluded, there was no difference in pre-operative PSV between adequate and inadequate fistulae and no increased failure rate with a PSV of <50cm/sec [7]. Therefore, above an arterial diameter of 2mm, arterial flow and PSV may be unimportant in determining fistula outcome.

Reactive hyperaemia

Ultimately, the best predictor of subsequent fistula maturation may be the ability to increase arterial inflow. Some women seem unable to increase PSV during the clenched fist manoeuvre and AV fistulae created in these patients have a poor outcome [7]. Interestingly, a failure to increase PSV during reactive hyperaemia did not influence outcome in men.

The RI is another potential measure of the artery to dilate. As diastolic flow increases in the hyperaemic state, the RI should fall. In one study [3], 95% of AV fistulae were successful if the hyperaemic RI of the feeding artery was less than 0.7, but only 39% when the hyperaemic RI was greater than 0.7. In another report, which excluded arteries <2mm in diameter there was no difference in the pre-operative hyperaemic RI between inadequate and adequate fistulae, so the potential to dilate may only be important in small arteries [7].

Venous diameter

Venous diameter is an important determinant of fistula outcome. In a prospective study, the mean cephalic vein diameters were significantly smaller in non-functioning AV fistulae (1.8 versus 2.2mm) [8]. In another report, a minimum pre-operative forearm cephalic vein diameter of <2.6mm predicted fistula failure in women but not in men [9]. In a further study of pre-operative vein mapping, successful maturation of wrist fistulae was significantly higher if the cephalic vein diameter was greater than 2.0mm [10]. Although a precise threshold has not been established, a minimum venous diameter (with a tourniquet) of 2.5mm is usually advised for AV fistulae, and 4.0mm for synthetic grafts [5].

The ability of a vein to dilate is an important predictor of success. Veins were found to dilate by 48% with a tourniquet in successful fistulae, compared with only 12% in fistulae that subsequently failed [11].

Evidence for the effectiveness of pre-operative ultrasound

A number of studies in the US have evaluated the impact of pre-operative ultrasound on the utilisation of native AV fistulae. Ultrasound is especially useful in the evaluation of obese patients in whom superficial veins are impalpable. These studies defined minimal requirements for a distal native AV fistula. Most require a distal radial artery diameter of 2mm or greater with a normal waveform and patent palmar arch, as well as a cephalic vein of 2.5mm or larger throughout its course to the subclavian vein. There must be no segmental stenosis or occlusion. Drainage of the cephalic vein into a large (>2.5mm) forearm medial cubital vein and brachial or basilic vein is also acceptable. The ipsilateral central veins must be normal. A prosthetic graft is recommended only if the outflow vein is greater than or equal to 4.0mm. Measurements of volume flow, peak systolic velocities or changes in RI following reactive hyperaemia are not routinely performed.

In a US study, routine pre-operative ultrasound significantly increased the prevalence of native access from 14% to 63%, reduced the early failure rate of native AV fistulae from 36% to 8.3% and increased the primary patency at one year from 48% to 83% in comparison with historical controls. As a result of the increased use of native AV access, the prevalence of prosthetic AV access reconstruction, as well as probable AV access complications, decreased significantly [5]. In another report the proportion of native fistulae increased from 34% in the historical control period to 64% with pre-operative mapping [12].

In a randomised prospective study, the rate of primary non-function was 5.6% with duplex ultrasound compared with 25% in patients undergoing only physical examination [13]. No long-term follow-up data were recorded. In another prospective study from the US, all patients underwent duplex mapping but the surgeon documented the planned access procedure based on physical examination results before reviewing the ultrasound report. Pre-operative ultrasound mapping resulted in a change to the planned surgical procedure in 31%. Native fistulae were placed in 58% of patients compared with 32% in a historical control period when mapping was not performed. Furthermore, no patient underwent unnecessary exploration of the arm [14].

These studies provide strong evidence for the routine use of pre-operative duplex scanning, which may become routine for screening prior to AV fistula formation. However, departments offering duplex scanning are often overstretched and it can be argued that with limited resources, scanning may not add to the assessment of straightforward cases with good pulses and adjacent veins. In a recent British study, the surgeon assessed patients clinically and a decision was made as to whether further pre-operative ultrasound investigation would be needed before fistula creation. All patients then underwent duplex ultrasound mapping. Ultrasound only altered the planned procedure in 1% (1/106) of cases in which imaging was deemed unnecessary compared to 50% (18/39) of cases where the clinical findings were unclear. This suggests that patients with good pulses and clinically adequate veins may proceed to surgery without pre-operative ultrasound mapping [15]. If duplex mapping is used routinely, it must not delay surgery.

Vessel mapping may also be useful for pre-operative planning in patients already receiving dialysis when the fistula or graft is failing [16].

Venography

For many years contrast venography was the gold standard imaging investigation prior to AV fistula formation. It has the particular advantage of providing a venous map, which many surgeons find useful. According to DOQI [1] , venography is mandatory in patients with a history of ipsilateral central vein catheterisation, collateral vein development, oedema or unilateral arm swelling, as these features may indicate central vein obstruction. Construction of a peripheral fistula in these patients can cause massive arm swelling and poor dialysis.

Until recently, temporary dialysis catheters were frequently placed in the subclavian veins causing a high incidence of venous stenosis. Today, best practice is to establish an AV fistula before commencing dialysis and, if this is not possible, insert a tunnelled right internal jugular line. This has reduced the incidence of central vein stenosis, although innominate vein stenosis remains a significant problem (Figure 3).

Venography with iodinated contrast is relatively contraindicated in pre-dialysis patients, as contrast nephropathy may precipitate acute renal failure. Duplex ultrasound is an alternative but is poor at assessing central vein stenosis. Contrast-enhanced MR venography has emerged as a promising alternative as the small volume of paramagnetic contrast agent used does not compromise renal function. A technique similar to conventional venography is used with contrast injected upstream of the

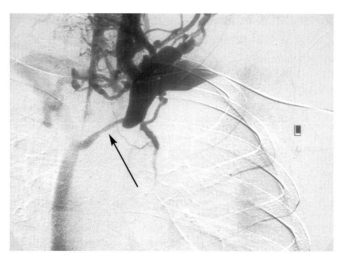

Figure 3 Venogram showing left innominate vein stenosis (arrow) due to a previous left internal jugular temporary dialysis line.

venous territory to be evaluated (Figure 4). To avoid T2 shortening effects the paramagnetic contrast should be diluted by a factor in the range 1: 10-20. Non-contrast MRI using time of flight (TOF) techniques have also been evaluated for pre-operative venous mapping, as there is also no risk of compromising renal function. Patients are examined prone with the arm under investigation inserted into a surface coil. The technique can be used successfully for venous mapping of the distal upper arm, elbow, and forearm with veins larger than 2mm visualised. The main limitation of the non-contrast technique is the inability to demonstrate proximal veins and venous distension.

In a prospective study comparing TOF MR venography and conventional venography prior to fistula formation, the demonstration of superficial veins and assessment of venous diameter were well correlated, and surgical findings correlated better with MR venography than conventional venography [17]. These results are encouraging but more data are needed before MR venographic techniques can be recommended for routine pre-operative evaluation.

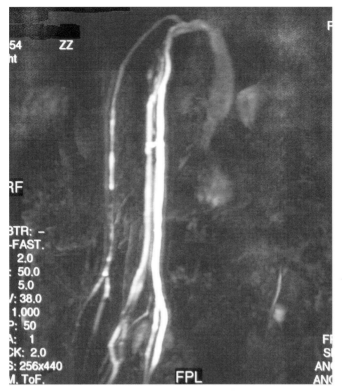

Figure 4 A contrast-enhanced MR venogram of the right upper arm.

Two further venographic techniques are available for the assessment of pre-dialysis patients without compromising renal function. Carbon dioxide (CO_2) venography has been used successfully to visualise both peripheral and central veins but has significant drawbacks, including local pain during injection, overestimation of venous stenoses and the risk of potentially serious complications, for example, acute right heart failure. A costly special injector may also be required. Despite these drawbacks CO_2 venography is widely used in several centres, particularly in France.

MRI contrast agents have also been evaluated using conventional X-ray digital subtraction techniques rather than magnetic resonance. Gadolinium-based contrast agents have shown they absorb sufficient energy to be visualised during angiography by digital subtraction.

However, the innominate veins and superior vena cava are relatively poorly visualised, which may limit the introduction of this technique.

Conclusions

Pre-operative imaging is effective at reducing the primary failure rate of AV fistulae and grafts. Ultrasound is effective at selecting target vessels and is readily available. If ultrasound is used routinely, surgery should not be delayed. Venography is still required to assess central vein stenosis. If iodinated contrast is contraindicated, MR venography is emerging as a suitable alternative.

Key Summary

◆ There is increasing evidence that routine pre-operative duplex ultrasound reduces the rate of primary fistula failure and unnecessary surgical exploration.

◆ Ultrasound increases the utilisation of native AV fistulae and allows proper selection of suitable target vessels of adequate diameter.

◆ A minimum arterial diameter of 2mm is associated with successful fistula formation. Below this diameter the ability of an artery to increase flow and dilate will determine fistula success.

◆ A threshold for minimal venous diameter is difficult to establish. Most clinical studies use a value of 2.5mm for AV fistulae and 4mm for prosthetic grafts (with a tourniquet).

◆ Traditional contrast venography is still an essential investigation if there is suspicion of central vein stenosis. In pre-dialysis patients MR venography is emerging as a suitable alternative.

References

1. The Vascular Access Work Group. NKF-DOQI clinical practice guidelines for vascular access. *Am J Kidney Dis* 1997; 30(suppl 3): S150-191.

2. Wong V, Ward R, Taylor J, *et al.* Factors associated with early failure of arteriovenous fistulae for haemodialysis access. *Eur J Vasc Endovasc Surg* 1996; 12: 207-13.

3. Malovrh M. Non-invasive evaluation of vessels by duplex sonography prior to construction of arteriovenous fistulas for haemodialysis. *Nephrol Dial Transplant* 1998; 13: 125-9.

4. Lemson MS, Leunissen KM, Tordoir JH. Does pre-operative duplex examination improve patency rates of Brescio-Cimino fistulas? *Nephrol Dial Transplant* 1998; 13: 1360-1.

5. Silva MB, Hobson RW, Pappas PJ, *et al.* A strategy for increasing use of autogenous hemodialysis access procedures: impact of preoperative non-invasive evaluation. *J Vasc Surg* 1998; 27: 302-8.

6. Sedlacek M, Teodorescue V, Falk A, *et al.* Hemodialysis access placement with pre-operative non-invasive vascular mapping: comparison between patients with and without diabetes. *Am J Kidney Dis* 2001; 38: 560-4

7. Lockhart ME, Robbin ML, Allon M. Pre-operative sonographic radial artery evaluation and correlation with subsequent radiocephalic fistula outcome. *J Ultrasound Med* 2004; 23: 161-8.

8. Tordoir JHM, Rooyens P, Dammers R, *et al.* Prospective evaluation of failure modes in autogenous radiocephalic wrist access for haemodialysis. *Nephrol Dial Transplant* 2003; 18: 378-83.

9. Brimble KS, Rabbat ChG, Treleavan DJ, *et al.* Utility of ultrasonographic venous assessment prior to forearm arteriovenous fistula creation. *Clin Nephrol* 2002; 58: 122-8.

10. Mendes RR, Farber MA, Marston WA, *et al.* Prediction of wrist arteriovenous fistula maturation with pre-operative vein mapping with ultrasonography. *J Vasc Surg* 2002; 36: 460-3.

11. Malovrh M. The role of sonography in the planning of arteriovenous fistulas for hemodialysis. *Semin Dial* 2003; 16(4): 229-303.

12. Allon M, Lockhart ME, Lilly RZ, *et al.* Effect of pre-operative sonographic mapping on vascular access outcomes in hemodialysis patients. *Kidney Int* 2001; 60: 2013-20.

13. Mihmanli I, Besirli K, Kurugoglu S, *et al.* Cephalic vein and hemodialysis fistula. *J Ultrasound Med* 2001; 20: 217-22.

14. Robbin M, Gallichio MH, Deierhoi MH, *et al.* US vascular mapping before hemodialysis access placement. *Radiology* 2000; 217: 83-8.

15. Wells AC, Fernando B, Butler A, *et al.* Selective use of ultrasonographic vascular mapping in the assessment of patients before haemodialysis access surgery. *Br J Surg* 2005; 92: 1439-43.

16. Jackson J, Litchfield TF. How a dedicated vascular access center can promote increased use of fistulas. *Nephrology Nursing Journal* 2006; 33: 189-96.

17.   Menegazzo D, Laissy J-P, Dürrbach, *et al*. Hemodialysis fistula creation: pre-operative assessment with MR venography and comparison with conventional venography. *Radiology* 1998; 209: 723-8.

Chapter 6

Primary access for haemodialysis

Christopher P Gibbons MA DPhil MCh FRCS

Consultant Surgeon, Morriston Hospital, Swansea, UK

Principles of vascular access - historical perspectives

In order to achieve successful haemodialysis blood must be circulated through a dialysis machine at the rate of at least 300ml/minute from an accessible blood vessel. At the beginning of haemodialysis in the 1960s access was provided by the Scribner shunt, which was a plastic conduit, tied into a suitable artery and vein (usually the radial artery and cephalic vein or the posterior tibial artery and long saphenous vein), which passed out through the skin in a loop. The venous and arterial ends could be connected to the machine to allow blood to flow across the dialysis membrane. The Scribner shunt had the great advantage of being usable immediately in the acute situation but was subject to repeated episodes of thrombosis and infection.

The arteriovenous (AV) fistula at the wrist was introduced by Brescia and Cimino in 1966. This gave a high blood flow in the cephalic vein allowing dialysis between two needles inserted during each session. Infection and thrombosis rates were low but a period of several weeks was necessary for maturation before needling. However, the introduction of the double-lumen central venous catheter for acute haemodialysis access allowed the Scribner shunt to be abandoned for acute dialysis.

Subsequently, further AV fistula sites in the upper limb and AV prosthetic grafts increased the options for haemodialysis access.

Options for vascular access - why autogenous?

Whilst emergency access is almost universally by the double-lumen central venous catheter, several options exist for long-term haemodialysis access. It is generally accepted that an autogenous AV fistula is the best option, with the lowest infection and the highest primary patency rates but takes several weeks to mature. Prosthetic AV grafts can be needled earlier and have similar secondary patency but have higher revision rates and are subject to local and systemic sepsis. Cuffed central venous lines can be used immediately but frequently thrombose and have high infection rates with consequent increased mortality.

In the author's experience of over 1800 access procedures, prosthetic grafts are rarely necessary. In a recent audit, prosthetic grafts were the primary access in only 0.3% (3.6% of all procedures). The snuffbox fistula comprised 54% of all primary procedures (34% all cases), wrist fistulae 33% primary (34% overall) and brachial fistulae 12% of primary access (20% overall). In the US, prosthetic grafts are popular and are still performed in 50-70% of cases, despite the somewhat conservative recommendation of the K-DOQI guidelines that at least 50% of primary access surgery should be autogenous fistulae [1]. In contrast, European centres have much lower graft usage in the order of 10-25% [2].

The principles of access planning [3]

A considerable proportion of new patients requiring dialysis present acutely, and demand emergency placement of a double-lumen central venous catheter. However, those presenting with slowly deteriorating renal function allow the requirement for dialysis to be anticipated. In such patients, the timely construction of an AV fistula will avoid the use of central lines with the attendant risks of sepsis and permit the commencement of dialysis on a mature fistula. The K-DOQI guidelines recommend that where possible a fistula should be constructed when the creatinine clearance is <25ml/minute or within 12 months of the anticipated need for dialysis [1]. UK guidelines advise the creation of vascular access 16-24 weeks before the predicted start of dialysis [4].

The primary considerations for an AV fistula are patency and ease of needling, but the preservation of other access sites is also important. The non-dominant upper limb is preferred so that the patient can perform self-needling for home dialysis or write and perform other tasks whilst dialysing. The most distal site is used first, moving proximally, depending on the availability of good veins and disease-free arteries.

Preservation of veins

It is essential to preserve upper limb veins in patients with renal failure. Intravenous cannulae should only be introduced if essential to treatment. Intravenous infusions should be restricted to the dorsum of the hand (preferably the dominant limb) or, failing this, the small veins on the palmar aspect of the wrist. The cephalic vein and veins in the antecubital fossa should be avoided completely, except in life-threatening situations demanding emergency access to the circulation. Once an AV fistula has been created it should be reserved exclusively for dialysis.

Fistula configurations - end-to-side or side-to-side?

In the original description of the AV fistula, a side-to-side configuration was advocated. However, distal venous flow is rarely significant and the increased risk of distal venous hypertension with ulceration with side-to-side fistulae led most surgeons to prefer the end-of-vein to side-of-artery configuration.

In radiocephalic AV fistulae, up to a third of fistula flow is retrograde from the distal artery. Occasionally this causes distal ischaemia (steal syndrome) leading some to advocate an end-to-end anastomosis (proximal artery to proximal vein) for radiocephalic AV fistulae. However, steal is infrequent and easily treated by distal arterial ligation so this configuration is rarely used [3].

Pre-operative investigation

In general, patients with visible upper limb veins and easily palpable pulses may proceed directly to surgery without further investigation. It is standard advice to perform an Allen test (observation of the capillary refill in the hand with the radial artery occluded) to check that the ulnar circulation is adequate, but there is little evidence that it is necessary in practice. If doubt exists regarding the arterial pulses or if a previous fistula has failed, a pre-operative duplex scan may help select the level for the fistula. If any significant (>70%) upstream arterial stenosis is suspected on Doppler examination, arteriography and angioplasty may be required.

Selective duplex mapping of the superficial veins in the presence of a tourniquet can also be helpful in patients with poorly visible veins, such as the obese, and in patients with previously failed access. Some units perform routine duplex vein mapping but the available evidence suggests that a selective policy is reasonable [5].

Duplex Doppler examination or venography of the subclavian and axillary veins should be performed if there is any limb swelling or venous collateral development around the shoulder and has been advocated as routine if a subclavian catheter has been used for acute dialysis [1].

Anaesthetic considerations

The majority of vascular access surgery is easily accomplished under local anaesthetic, although some surgeons prefer an axillary block believing that the vasodilatation produced is beneficial for access patency, but there is no hard evidence to support this. Up to 75% of patients can be treated as day cases. In the author's unit dialysis access surgery is performed almost exclusively on a dedicated local anaesthetic list. An anaesthetist is not required but an anaesthetic nurse is a great advantage to provide close monitoring and administer prophylactic antibiotics (usually cefuroxime 750mg i.v.) and sedation (diazepam 5-10mg i.v.). Blood pressure, ECG, and pulse oximetry are continuously monitored and 28% oxygen is given routinely by mask. For most procedures 10-20ml 0.5% bupivacaine or laevo-bupivacaine by local infiltration provides adequate anaesthesia. When the operation is extended, for instance to a forearm vein loop or PTFE loop, further bupivacaine or laevo-bupivacaine 0.25% can be injected.

Surgical options

The snuffbox AV fistula (Figure 1)

The most distal AV fistula site is between the cephalic vein and the radial artery in the anatomical snuffbox [5, 6]. This is the preferred fistula in the author's unit [6] and can be constructed in approximately 50% of new dialysis patients, although the smaller vessels of women make them less ideal and give poorer patencies. The overall patency is similar to classical Brescia-Cimino wrist fistulae, which can still be performed in about 45% of failed snuffbox fistulae.

A 3-4cm longitudinal incision over the anatomical snuffbox gives access to the underlying cephalic vein and following further infiltration of anaesthetic beneath the extensor retinaculum the distal radial artery is exposed. Larger arterial branches are divided between 4/0 vicryl ties, whereas small branches may be coagulated with bipolar diathermy and divided to mobilise an adequate length of vessel. Control is obtained using atraumatic microvascular clamps such as Scovill-Lewis or Yasargil.

The cephalic vein is divided distally, after ligating with 4/0 vicryl, spatulated and flushed with heparinised Ringers containing papaverine (4mg/l). An end-to-side anastomosis is then fashioned using 6/0 polypropylene with an 8mm needle. Non-penetrating vascular clips can be used for the anastomosis instead of sutures, provided the vessels are not calcified and there is evidence from randomised trials that they improve patency [6, 7]. A successful fistula demonstrates a palpable thrill, whereas a pulse in the vein without a thrill indicates a downstream venous stenosis and imminent failure. If the fistula thromboses rapidly it may be reopened and thrombectomised, but in the author's experience a technical reason for failure is rarely found and the fistula usually fails again. Postoperatively, the arm is warmed in a Gamgee sleeve to promote vasodilatation.

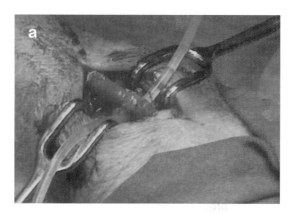

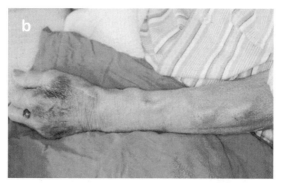

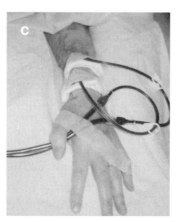

Figure 1 The snuffbox AV fistula: a) prior to closure; b) the mature fistula; c) in use showing the distal needle placement.

The radiocephalic AV fistula at the wrist (Figure 2)

When the cephalic vein is poor distally or the radial pulse is not palpable in the anatomical snuffbox, the standard AV fistula at the wrist is the next option [3, 6, 8]. The author's preference is an oblique or sigmoid incision under local anaesthetic to allow an end-to-side anastomosis. A radiocephalic AV fistula can also be performed at almost any site in the forearm, although the radial artery becomes progressively deeper in the upper forearm and access becomes slightly more difficult. The brachio-radialis tendon overlies the radial artery above the wrist and requires partial division to provide adequate access and avoid kinking of the cephalic vein as it is brought down to anastomose to the radial artery.

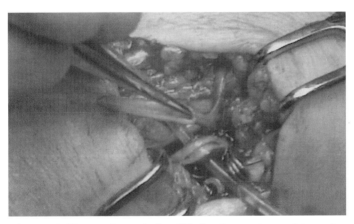

Figure 2 The radiocephalic AV fistula at the wrist under construction, showing the mobilisation of the vein (superiorly with forceps in lumen) to reach the radial arteriotomy.

The brachial AV fistula (Figure 3)

If good forearm veins are unavailable most patients are suitable for a fistula in the antecubital fossa [9]. Local anaesthetic (10-15ml 0.5% bupivacaine) is again used, infiltrating the skin and subcutaneous tissue to permit a transverse incision to expose the superficial veins. After further deep anaesthetic infiltration the deep fascia and bicipital aponeurosis are

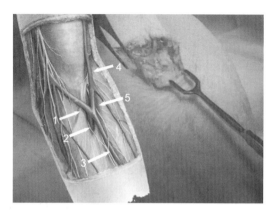

a) Venous exposure with most common venous anatomy inset:

1 median basilic vein;
2 deep perforating vein;
3 distal cephalic vein;
4 proximal cephalic vein;
5 median cephalic vein.

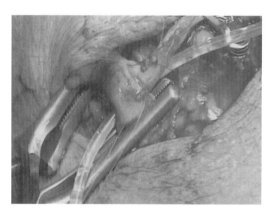

b) End-to-side anastomosis of median cephalic vein to brachial artery.

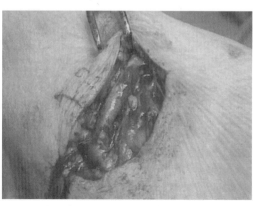

c) Completed fistula.

Figure 3 The brachiocephalic AV fistula.

divided to expose the brachial artery, which can be isolated over a suitable length for anastomosis. In the occasional patient with a high bifurcation of the brachial artery, either the radial or ulnar arteries can be used for the anastomosis.

The venous anatomy is variable and in some cases this may be compounded by thrombosis due to previous intravenous infusions. There are several anastomotic possibilities:

- the first choice is an end-to-side brachiocephalic AV fistula using the median cephalic vein;
- an alternative is to use the deep perforating vein if it will reach the artery without tension (the Gracz fistula);
- in some cases the median cephalic vein is thrombosed and the proximal cephalic vein itself can be mobilised to reach the brachial artery;
- when the cephalic vein is unusable an AV fistula can be constructed to the median basilic vein but this gives only a short length of usable vein. This may be suitable for single-needle, or occasionally, double-needle dialysis and is worth trying. If dialysis proves problematical the fistula can be later converted to a basilic vein transposition;
- where no superficial veins are available but the vein accompanying the brachial artery is adequate, a prosthetic AV loop can be constructed in the forearm following further local anaesthetic infiltration (0.25% or 0.5% laevo-bupivacaine).

Other options

Where the radial artery or cephalic vein is unusable, an ulnobasilic AV fistula can be constructed in the forearm or wrist under local anaesthesia. The basilic vein is usually disease-free as it is rarely used for intravenous infusions but the resultant fistula is difficult to needle.

In a few patients the forearm arteries are diseased but the veins are good. In such cases the cephalic (or basilic) vein can be dissected out through a longitudinal incision and looped back in a subcutaneous tunnel to anastomose to the brachial artery forming a forearm vein loop. In other cases, the basilic vein can be mobilised and brought subcutaneously across the anterior forearm to join the radial artery or the cephalic vein brought across similarly to the ulnar artery.

Finally, fistulae between a tibial artery and the long saphenous vein have been reported where the upper limbs are completely unusable.

Problem patients

Obesity

Patients, especially women, with obese arms and little in the way of visible veins can provide a difficult challenge. It is often worth exploring the wrist, for in many cases a reasonable cephalic vein is found and can be used to create a wrist or snuffbox fistula. The vein can be superficialised by defatting the overlying skin for a few centimetres proximally giving a sufficient length for needling. This may be enhanced by weight loss, which often occurs when dialysis commences. In others a brachiocephalic fistula may be possible as the fat layer is often thin in the antecubital fossa, but a prosthetic forearm AV graft may be required in some cases.

Poor veins

Patients who have had multiple hospital admissions and operations may have had multiple intravenous infusions. This is particularly frequent in poorly controlled insulin-dependent diabetics who may have had hypertonic glucose infusions. In such cases the upper limb veins have often thrombosed. Vein mapping may be helpful to choose the correct level for a fistula in this situation. However, there is no easy answer to such difficult patients and the most distal autogenous fistula should be performed, although disappointment may ensue when two or more attempts may be needed to achieve satisfactory function.

Calcified arteries

In some cases, particularly diabetics, the distal arteries are calcified. In some cases with mild calcification bulldog clamps can achieve arterial control and the vessel will hold sutures; other options include the use of an occlusion balloon or a proximal tourniquet. In others an anastomosis is impossible and a more proximal fistula, usually brachial, is required.

Proximal arterial disease

If the distal pulses are poor or a first fistula fails an arterial duplex Doppler should be performed and will detect any proximal arterial stenosis. Pre-operative angioplasty may then permit a successful fistula.

Subclavian vein thrombosis

Upper limb oedema often indicates a subclavian or innominate vein stenosis or occlusion, but in many cases pain and swelling only becomes apparent after the fistula becomes functional. Subclavian angioplasty or stenting will settle the oedema and allow fistula formation, but recurrence of the venous obstruction is common.

Complications [2, 3]

Bleeding

Bleeding is remarkably rare after autogenous AV fistula creation, despite the platelet dysfunction associated with renal failure. Persistent oozing from small cutaneous vessels occurs occasionally and can usually be stopped by intradermal injection of 1 or 2% lignocaine with adrenaline. If this fails an extra suture may be required.

Infection

Infection usually responds to antibiotics but occasionally severe sepsis may cause severe haemorrhage requiring fistula ligation.

Thrombosis

Thrombosis is the most common complication. For early thrombosis some surgeons return the patient to theatre for thrombectomy as an emergency. The author has not found this to be worthwhile as rethrombosis is frequent. It is better to accept failure and create a new fistula at a higher level on the next available list after a duplex scan. If local expertise exists, radiological intervention by thrombolysis and angioplasty may salvage a fistula after late failure but the author's preference is to form a new fistula under local anaesthetic at the earliest opportunity.

Steal

Steal is rare in distal AV fistulae but occasionally thumb ulceration or necrosis indicates radial steal. The measurement of thumb pressure by a small cuff and photoplethysmography confirms ischaemia, which can be normalised by compression of the distal radial artery. Distal radial artery ligation will cure the problem in most cases but fistula ligation is occasionally necessary. Brachial fistulae may cause more severe ischaemia of the hand ranging from rest pain to digital gangrene. Ligation of the fistula cures the problem but destroys the access. Banding the fistula with careful intra-operative pressure measurements, the DRIL procedure (distal arterial ligation with interval revascularisation), preferably with intra-operative needle pressure measurements, or dismantling the fistula and extending the vein onto the radial artery 2-3cm from the origin (the extension procedure) will usually cure the problem and preserve the fistula (see Chapter 10).

Aneurysm

Many fistulae become aneurysmal with time but few require treatment. However, where rupture appears imminent there is usually little option other than to ligate the fistula and create another one at a more proximal site, although short aneurysmal segments may be bypassed using saphenous vein.

High output cardiac failure

High output cardiac failure is an occasional problem with brachial fistulae and may require fistula revision or ligation.

Results of primary access

In general 10% of autogenous fistulae will thrombose in the first few hours and a further 10% will either thrombose or fail to develop adequately for use within six weeks. Primary patencies of 60-70% at one year and 40-50% at five years are usual [10]. Prosthetic AV grafts have similar secondary patency but revision rates of several times that of autogenous fistulae. Infection rates and associated mortality are considerably lower for autogenous fistulae than either prosthetic grafts or central venous catheters.

Factors affecting patency [2, 8]

Thrombosis is the commonest cause of access failure. It may be precipitated by hypercoagulable states, for instance during surgery or intercurrent illness and is more common in smokers. Traumatic needling with haematoma formation and subsequent fibrosis may result in a venous stenosis and fistula thrombosis. However, in many cases a stenosis due to intimal hyperplasia of the vein is the ultimate cause of failure. Access surveillance by various techniques may detect such stenoses and allow their correction prior to thrombosis (see Chapter 12). Thrombosis is commoner in women, and in patients with small vessels or poor fistula flow. Diabetes has been an adverse factor for patency in some studies but not others. Whilst there is remarkably little evidence from randomised trials, antiplatelet agents such as aspirin and dipyridamole probably prolong fistula patency and are used routinely in most units. Warfarin is recommended in patients with hypercoagulable states. A glyceryl trinitrate patch over the venous outflow reduces the thrombophlebitis associated with intravenous infusions and may also improve initial fistula patency, but this needs to be proven in randomised trials. The improved haemoglobin levels with the increasing use of erythropoietin in end-stage renal failure might be expected to reduce access patency but evidence from randomised trials suggests that this is not the case.

Needling strategies [6]

For most fistulae a maturation period of 4-6 weeks is required to allow arterialisation of the venous outflow. An experienced dialysis nurse should perform initial needling as the fistula is at its most vulnerable to extravasation of blood, which can lead to perivascular fibrosis and stenosis. Cannulation can be performed using one of three strategies (Figure 4):

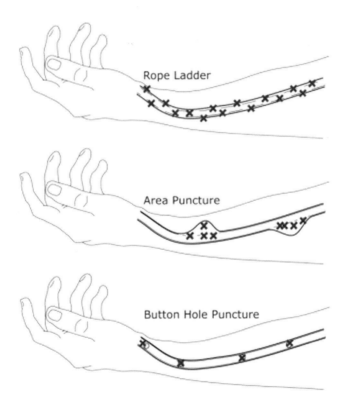

Figure 4 Needling strategies for AV fistulae.

- Rope ladder. Systematic evenly spaced cannulation along the length of the vein causes mild and evenly distributed dilatation and is more suited to prosthetic grafts.
- Area puncture. Repeated puncture over short segments of vein encourages dilatation in a new fistula but sometimes causes interspersed stenoses.
- Buttonhole. Repeated puncture through the same site causes little dilatation but reduces pain.

Conclusions

It is possible to construct an autogenous AV fistula in the vast majority of patients requiring haemodialysis access. Distal fistulae have many advantages including ease of needling, reduced infection rates and preservation of proximal sites, although the lower flow rates than with proximal fistulae or prosthetic grafts sometimes necessitate longer dialysis times. In the author's unit, less than 2% of patients are currently dialysing on prosthetic fistulae.

The major problem facing nephrologists and surgeons is the rapidly increasing dialysis population. Surgeons are finding it increasingly difficult to keep up with demand. A dedicated vascular access list (which can be a local anaesthetic list in the day-case theatre) is essential. In the past, many vascular surgeons have failed to take an interest in access surgery, but with the expansion of dialysis units outside transplant centres vascular surgeons have become pivotal in ensuring that dialysis is maintained in those patients requiring renal replacement therapy.

Key Summary

◆ In patients with renal failure, forearm and upper arm veins must be preserved for dialysis access and should not be used for venepunctures or intravenous cannulae.

◆ Primary vascular access should be an autogenous AV fistula in the vast majority of patients.

◆ The most distal fistula possible should be performed preferably in the non-dominant upper limb.

◆ Pre-operative duplex scanning is useful in patients with failed fistulae, uncertain arterial status or patients at risk of subclavian venous occlusion.

◆ Local anaesthetic is adequate for most patients.

◆ Complications of distal autogenous fistulae are rare except for thrombosis, which occurs in up to 20% in the first six weeks.

◆ Steal syndromes are more common with proximal fistulae.

◆ Fistula patency is poorer in women and patients with narrow veins.

◆ Antiplatelet agents probably improve fistula patency.

References

1.   NKF-K/DOQI Clinical Practice Guidelines for Vascular Access: Update 2000. *Am J Kidney Dis* 2001; 37(1) Suppl 1: S137-81.

2.   Allon M, Robbin ML. Increasing arteriovenous fistulas in hemodialysis patients: problems and solutions. *Kidney Int* 2002; 62: 1109-24.

3.   Nicholson ML, Murphy GJ. Surgical considerations in vascular access. In: *Haemodialysis Vascular Access: Practice and Problems.* Conlon PJ, Schwab SJ, Nicholson ML, Eds. Oxford: Oxford University Press, 2000: 101-23.

4.   Winearls CG, Fluck R, Mitchell DC, *et al.* The organization and delivery of the vascular access service for maintenance haemodialysis patients. Report of a joint working party. 2006. http://www.vascularsociety.org.uk/Docs/VASCULAR%20ACCESS%20JOINT%20WORKING%20PARTY%20REPORT.pdf.

5.   Wells AC, Fernando B, Butler A, *et al.* Selective use of ultrasonographic vascular mapping in the assessment of patients before haemodialysis access surgery. *Br J Surg* 2005; 92: 1439-43.

6.   Andrew J, Gibbons CP. Vascular access for haemodialysis. In: *Pathways of Care in Vascular Surgery.* Beard JD, Murray S, Eds. Shrewsbury, UK: tfm Publishing Ltd, 2002: 241-54.

7.   Shenoy S, Miller A, Petersen F, *et al.* A multicentre study of permanent hemodialysis access patency: beneficial effect of clipped vascular anastomotic technique. *J Vasc Surg* 2003; 38: 229-35.

8.   Gibbons CP. Haemodialysis access. In: *The Evidence for Vascular Surgery,* 2nd Ed. Earnshaw JJ, Murie JA, Eds. Shrewsbury, UK: tfm Publishing Ltd, 2006: 117-8.

9.   Nicholson ML, Polo JR. Upper arm arteriovenous fistulas. In: *Haemodialysis Vascular Access: Practice and Problems.* Conlon PJ, Schwab SJ, Nicholson ML, Eds. Oxford: Oxford University Press, 2000: 123-40.

10.   Rooijens PP, Tordoir JH, Stijnen T, *et al.* Radiocephalic wrist arteriovenous fistula for hemodialysis: meta-analysis indicates a high primary failure rate. *Eur J Vasc Endovasc Surg* 2004; 28: 583-9.

Chapter 7
Tertiary vascular access

David C Mitchell MA MB MS FRCS

Consultant Vascular & Transplant Surgeon, Southmead Hospital, Bristol, UK

Introduction

The procedure of choice for primary vascular access is the Brescia-Cimino wrist fistula, fashioned by joining the end of the divided cephalic vein to the side of the radial artery. If this fails, it is usual to perform secondary procedures between the same artery and vein at varying levels in the forearm or in the antecubital fossa. Tertiary access procedures are those that follow the failure of both primary and secondary procedures. This chapter provides an overview of the principles guiding choice of permanent access for patients with failed wrist and brachial arteriovenous (AV) fistulae. Central venous catheters are usually required while awaiting fistula maturation but also may be indicated in the longer term for some patients where a satisfactory fistula cannot be established. They are considered in Chapter 4.

Principles of tertiary access

General patient characteristics must be considered. It is important to exclude general causes of fistula failure, such as persistent hypotension, or a systemic pre-disposition to thrombosis. These may compromise any subsequent procedure and should be addressed at the outset. Untreated cardiac failure and septicaemia are contraindications to fistula surgery. Persistent hypotension due to the selection of an inappropriately low 'dry' weight of a dialysis patient may require correction by pre-operative rehydration and patients with inherited thrombotic tendencies may require anticoagulation. Using the patient's own veins is the best way to achieve a durable fistula. Autogenous AV fistulae may be more difficult to establish, but require much less revision (about once in every eight years) than synthetic grafts (80% require revision within a year) [1, 2]. In some cases, durability may be less important than the ease of surgery. The fistula of choice may then be a synthetic AV bridge graft.

In a patient with a previously failed access, a systematic approach is required. The principles are to identify appropriate sites for further access and to plan procedures that conserve veins for the future. It is important not to overlook the possibility of straightforward fistula creation before embarking on more demanding and complex procedures.

Venous assessment

Autogenous AV fistulae may still be fashioned, despite the failure of forearm AV fistulae. Sometimes simple clinical examination may reveal suitable veins, but often, particularly in the obese, adequate veins cannot be found. Some form of pre-operative imaging is often required to assess the adequacy of the upper limb veins. The author prefers duplex ultrasound for this, measuring the diameter of the major veins with the arm dependent or a proximal tourniquet [3]. Venography is an alternative and may be required if the central veins cannot be imaged with ultrasound. Bilateral upper limb venograms can give a wealth of information, establishing both the size and patency of the veins and the presence or absence of central vein stenosis.

Central venous stenosis may follow the liberal use of central venous catheters, particularly subclavian lines, which are now avoided in most renal units. If untreated, central vein stenoses may contribute to fistula failure or to re-circulation and inefficient dialysis. Angioplasty of such lesions should be preferably performed before fistula surgery. Persistent arm swelling and venous engorgement may indicate a residual central venous stenosis requiring repeat angioplasty or stenting.

If the veins at the wrist are small, but of adequate calibre near the elbow, a prosthetic forearm loop graft is an option. A randomised controlled trial from The Netherlands has shown that such grafts can provide good quality access, albeit at the expense of a higher revision rate [4]. They may also encourage enlargement of arm veins, enabling conversion to an autogenous fistula following graft failure. Forearm loop grafts may be associated with lower rates of steal than brachial AV fistulae [5].

In the absence of suitable arm veins, the long saphenous vein may be imaged with duplex ultrasound. Thigh fistulae may provide a durable access, but the proximity of needling points to the groin, makes them more susceptible to infection. In addition, the arterial supply to the leg is more susceptible to atherosclerosis than the upper limb, especially in older and diabetic patients. Patients undergoing proximal limb fistula operations should be warned of the possibility of steal syndrome prior to surgery.

Arterial assessment

Pulse palpation may be all that is required in the fit younger patient. In others, especially in redo surgery and where the adequacy of the arterial circulation is uncertain, arterial duplex scanning can be helpful to exclude stenosis at sites of previous surgery and to assess the patency of distal vessels. Patients with persistent hypotension and diseased vessels are more likely to have poor fistula flow and suffer thrombosis. As patients with renal failure age, their arteries calcify and this may make ultrasound assessment difficult. Wrist fistulae are more prone to failure in elderly patients with diabetes [6], in whom proximal fistulae are more likely to succeed. A pragmatic approach is to use duplex scanning when there is uncertainty. The author prefers to use an artery of at least 2mm in diameter with a bi- or tri-phasic signal.

Types of tertiary access

Arteriovenous fistulae

Radiocephalic forearm fistulae
It is reasonable to attempt a further autogenous fistula if a good quality forearm vein and artery can be identified, despite previous failed access procedures. A further radiocephalic AV fistula is often feasible higher in the

forearm. Alternatives in the forearm include an ulnobasilic fistula (see Chapter 6) and the subcutaneous transposition of the basilic vein to the radial artery. It is advisable to warn the patient that the risk of failure may be greater than that of the primary procedure.

Upper arm AV fistulae

A brachiocephalic fistula in the antecubital fossa is the next choice. In the upper arm, more proximal brachiocephalic fistulae are difficult to fashion due to the increasing distance between artery and vein above the elbow.

Basilic vein transposition

Often a good-sized basilic vein can be identified. This vein is of great value as it lies deep within the limb, close to the artery and has usually been spared venesection. The vein can be mobilised through a medial arm incision, taking care to avoid the median cutaneous nerves of the arm and forearm. Having mobilised the vein to the level of the axilla, it is then tunnelled subcutaneously under the skin of the anterior surface of the arm, coming to lie adjacent to the brachial artery in the distal arm. An end-to-side anastomosis allows development of the vein, which if large can be used within a couple of weeks. This so-called basilic vein transposition AV fistula (Figure 1) is a very useful tertiary procedure in the younger patient where fistula durability may be at a premium. Success rates of 75% are quoted [7]. If the vein is of small calibre (less than 3mm) or the brachial artery diseased, it is possible to do a primary brachiobasilic AV fistula under local anaesthetic. If the fistula develops, then it can be secondarily transposed by dividing the vein at the anastomosis, tunnelling it subcutaneously over the biceps and re-anastomosing it more proximally to the brachial artery. Some surgeons advocate this two-stage procedure routinely.

Lower limb AV fistulae

If suitable vein cannot be found in the upper limb, then a thorough search of the lower limb is the next step. A long saphenous vein of more than 3.5mm in diameter can provide useful access, provided the arterial

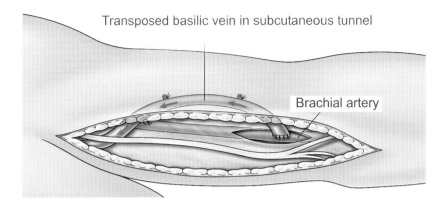

Transposed basilic vein in subcutaneous tunnel

Brachial artery

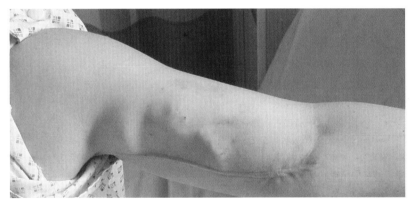

Figure 1 The basilic vein transposition fistula.

inflow is intact. The procedure of choice is a subcutaneous transposition of the vein onto the anterior thigh. This is performed through two incisions: oblique in the groin and vertical in the thigh, to expose and mobilise the vein. This is then tunnelled superficially and brought to lie over the distal superficial femoral artery. An end-to-side anastomosis completes the procedure. Such a straight configuration AV fistula is less likely to have technical problems than tunnelling the vein in a loop back to the groin.

When the long saphenous vein is absent or inadequate, the femoral vein can be transposed superficially and anastomosed to the superficial femoral artery in the thigh or looped back to the common femoral artery. The superficial femoral vein can also be excised and inserted as an AV graft in the arm. The large calibre of the superficial femoral vein makes it an excellent conduit but the resulting high flows give a considerable risk of distal ischaemia due to steal (see Chapter 10).

Prosthetic access grafts

Where no adequate vein exists, the surgeon should consider a synthetic arteriovenous bridge graft. The graft itself is punctured for dialysis. The usual prosthetic material is polytetrafluoroethylene (PTFE), but others such as polyurethane are available (see Chapter 8). However, it is not self-sealing so that prolonged compression may be required and repeated needling at the same site may lead to false aneurysm formation. Self-sealing grafts have been tried and may have needling advantages but seem to have poorer patency. Treated biomaterials such as bovine mesenteric vein and bovine ureter have also been used.

The requirements for a synthetic graft are a suitable arterial inflow and a vein to provide an adequate venous outflow. There is debate as to whether straight or looped configurations provide more durable access, but this remains unresolved [8]. For looped grafts, a central externally supported segment may prevent kinking. Stepped or tapered PTFE grafts which have a narrower arterial end to reduce flow and limit steal may be used in some circumstances.

A variety of anatomical graft configurations may be used in the upper limb (Figure 2), e.g. a straight radiobasilic graft, a brachiobasilic forearm loop or a brachio-axillary graft. For loop grafts the venae comitantes around the brachial artery are sometimes adequate for the venous anastomosis if no other vein is patent at the antecubital fossa. In the lower limb, a femorofemoral thigh loop is usually used but some advocate a straight graft between the superficial femoral or popliteal artery and the common femoral vein (Figures 3 and 4). In extreme situations, surgical ingenuity has led to unusual AV bridge graft configurations such as axillo-axillary grafts across the sternum or ilio-iliac or aorto-vena cava loops passing out through the abdominal wall to allow continued dialysis (see Chapter 9).

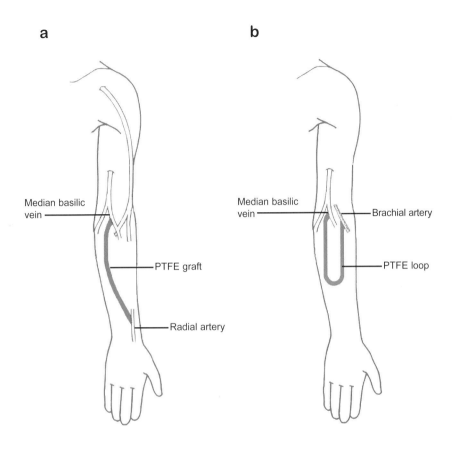

Figure 2 Forearm prosthetic grafts: a) straight radiobasilic configuration; b) brachiobasilic forearm loop.

Most grafts are relatively easy to establish and require a brief period of incorporation (7-10 days), rather than the several weeks of maturation required by an AV fistula. The disadvantage is that they are prone to infection and thrombosis. Infection can be reduced by rigorous asepsis during needling and by the eradication of nasal carriage of *Staphylococcus aureus* by topical agents such as mupirocin [9]. Thrombosis is usually due to intimal hyperplasia at the venous

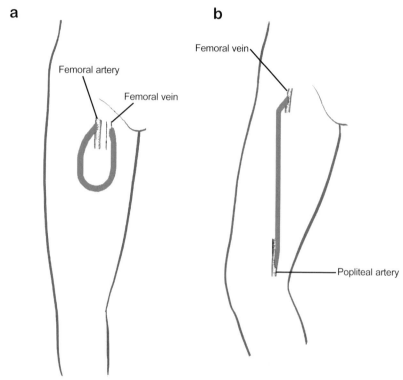

Figure 3 Prosthetic thigh AF fistulae: a) femorofemoral thigh loop; b) popliteal-femoral.

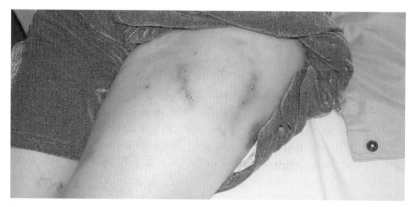

Figure 4 A patient with a femorofemoral prosthetic thigh loop.

anastomosis. If detected early, this can be dealt with by angioplasty (see Chapter 13), but once thrombosis intervenes, then a short extension graft to undamaged vein is often required. The addition of a venous cuff [10] or a wide expansion at the venous end of a PTFE graft may improve haemodynamics, reduce anastomotic intimal hyperplasia and, at least for the PTFE cuff, seems to improve patency in practice [11].

There are significant differences in graft usage throughout the world. This probably reflects cultural preference rather than racial differences in vessel quality. Most information on grafts comes from the US, whereas the data on AV fistulae are principally European in origin. There has been a debate as to the relative merits of fistulae and grafts. The National Kidney Foundation Dialysis Outcomes Quality Initiative (NKF-DOQI) [12] is a set of standards developed for the American healthcare market. It favours starting dialysis with a fistula, but falls short of advising against grafts. With adequate surveillance programs, graft patency approaches that of fistulae at the cost of a significantly greater number of interventions.

As prosthetic AV bridge grafts may be easier to establish, some clinicians favour them in the older patient, the obese and those with limited life expectancy where durability is not the primary concern. The choice of anaesthetic is usually a matter of personal preference, although in frail patients, a loco-regional block may be the technique of choice.

Central venous catheters

Whereas central venous catheters are mainly indicated for temporary access whilst awaiting placement of definitive access, for a small number of patients in whom a fistula or graft cannot be established, they may be used for long-term access. Catheters should ideally be placed in the internal jugular vein, as subclavian catheterisation may cause rapid fibrosis around the catheter and subclavian vein stenosis or occlusion. They should either be a tunnelled line, with a cuff to minimise sepsis, or a wholly implantable device that can be needled percutaneously for dialysis. These are dealt with more thoroughly in Chapter 4. With care, patients can be managed with lines for many years. The principal problems are thrombosis of the line, infection and fibrin cuff formation around the line impeding blood flow and making dialysis inefficient.

Catheter thrombosis and infection are best dealt with by removal and subsequent replacement of the line. When dialysis is required immediately, a line change may still resolve the problem. Fibrin cuff formation may be dealt with by percutaneous stripping of the fibrin cuff using interventional techniques [13], or by catheter thrombolysis [14], but changing the line over the wire may give superior patency [15]. If these strategies fail, rotating the line to a new site is advised.

Complications (see also Chapter 10)

Infection

Infection is a particular problem of foreign implanted material. Infection does occur in autogenous AV fistulae but they are much more resistant to sepsis than grafts or lines. Gross inflammation, abscess formation, rapidly expanding aneurysms and secondary haemorrhage are indications for moving to a new site. Otherwise, fistula-associated sepsis can be managed with high-dose antibiotics in the first instance. Infection in synthetic grafts or lines is likely in patients with fever and rigors, irrespective of blood culture results. If no source can be clearly identified, then prolonged antibiotics may solve the problem. If a line is present, then it should be removed and replaced once the septic episode is over. If the situation is desperate, then line changes under antibiotic cover can sometimes resolve the infection. In synthetic grafts, frank pus, widespread inflammation and secondary haemorrhage are indications for graft removal. Local resection and interposition grafting can occasionally deal with local abscess formation over a needle site in a well incorporated graft. This requires prolonged antibiotic administration and a clear understanding that early recurrence of sepsis is an indication for graft removal [9].

Thrombosis

This is common in the presence of stenosis. In grafts and now also autogenous fistulae there is evidence that surveillance prevents thrombosis and promotes long-term function [16-19] (see also Chapter 12). If routine intra-dialysis monitoring shows poor fistula function, then investigation by duplex ultrasound is reasonable. In the author's unit, flows of <500ml/min and a stenosis of >50% are an indication for revision. For a stenosis adjacent to the anastomosis, surgical revision with fistula ligation, division and proximal re-anastomosis is the best management. More remote stenoses are best managed with balloon angioplasty. It is the author's practice to rescan revised fistulae at six weeks to ensure improved function, although no evidence currently exists to support this approach.

There is debate about the use of antiplatelet agents and anticoagulants in grafts or AV fistulae that have previously thrombosed. The pragmatic approach is to anticoagulate those patients with particular thrombotic problems and those in whom alternative fistula sites are difficult to identify.

Steal syndrome

If the distal circulation is diseased, blood may flow preferentially into the fistula and be 'stolen' from the distal limb [20]. Large fistula flows are often seen in patients with steal. Steal syndrome is diagnosed by a cold pale extremity with poor or absent pulsation. Neurological symptoms of numbness, weakness, tingling and pain, may be associated with signs of motor or sensory deficit. Confirmation of steal is provided by manual occlusion of the fistula and return of normal perfusion to the extremity. Once diagnosed, treatment should follow without delay. Waiting more than a few hours may lead to permanent neurological injury and an ischaemic contracture. Often such fistulae have been fashioned in difficult circumstances. Simple fistula ligation is curative but destroys vital dialysis access. In this situation, the Distal Reconstruction and Interval Ligation (DRIL) procedure may salvage both fistula and limb [21]. An arterial bypass is fashioned from above to below the fistula. It is recommended that the inflow should be about 8cm above the fistula. The distal anastomosis should lie a few centimetres distal to the fistula. Once completed satisfactorily, the artery between the fistula and the distal anastomosis is occluded. If this returns normal blood flow and sensation to the extremity, then the artery is ligated, forcing flow down the bypass. The procedure works by diverting antegrade flow to the arm and by preventing retrograde flow from the distal artery to the fistula. In some cases simple arterial ligation distal to the fistula may solve the problem, by preventing retrograde flow and allowing the limb to be perfused through collateral channels. However, this should only be performed without bypass if intra-operative pressure measurements show that distal arterial pressure is adequate after ligation.

Alternatives include detaching the fistula from the brachial artery and extending the fistula onto the radial artery 2-3cm from its origin (the extension procedure) or reducing the flow by narrowing the draining vein over a short segment (banding) with the help of intra-operative flow measurements [22] (see Chapter 10).

Cardiac failure

High fistula flows can also cause high-output cardiac failure; this is seen more commonly in proximal AV fistulae and grafts. In these cases, fistula or graft revision is required to reduce flow. The choices include sacrificing the fistula and creating a new access, or attempting a flow reduction procedure. Banding the fistula controlling the procedure with intra-operative flow measurements, may work, but postoperative thrombosis is not uncommon. It is the author's preference to insert a short segment of 4mm or 5mm diameter PTFE graft into the fistula at or adjacent to the anastomosis, which seems to provide a more reliable way of controlling fistula flow. For brachial AV fistulae the extension procedure (see above) is an alternative.

Conclusions

Tertiary vascular access procedures are undertaken after initial attempts at access have failed. An AV fistula is the optimum, and can often be performed even after several previous failed access procedures. A prosthetic graft or a more complex procedure such as basilic vein transposition may be used if this is not feasible or the AV fistula fails. Thorough pre-operative vascular investigation should identify the ideal site for further access placement. Central lines can be used for temporary dialysis and also long-term dialysis in those patients in whom fistula or graft placement is not an option. Detailed discussion with the patient about the likelihood of success and potential complications is important.

Key Summary

◆ **Avoid central lines whenever possible.** Catheters cause fibrosis and narrowing of central veins. This may render the arm unsuitable for vascular access. Long-term use may be required if no fistula can be established.

◆ **AV fistulae rather than AV prosthetic grafts.** AV fistulae have better primary patency, require fewer interventions and have reduced infection rates than prosthetic bridge grafts.

◆ **Image veins prior to tertiary access.** Suitable veins can often be found. Central vein stenosis can be detected and treated to preserve access if needed.

◆ **Image arteries with duplex if there is any doubt about patency.** Diseased arteries predispose to steal syndrome. Poor arterial inflow can jeopardise success in the elderly and in diabetics.

◆ **Consent.** Warn of possibility of further failure. In established proximal AV fistulae in the elderly and diabetics, warn of steal (up to 8%) and cardiac failure. Synthetic grafts have an 80% chance of needing revision within a year in comparison with 12-15% for autogenous fistulae.

◆ **Complications.** Infection and thrombosis are the biggest problems. Skip grafts may work for localised graft exposure or sepsis, but an abscess along the length of the graft, or secondary haemorrhage from the anastomosis, is an absolute indication for removal. If steal is diagnosed, urgent revision (ligation, DRIL procedure or banding) is required to avoid permanent neurological injury.

References

1. Pisoni RL, Young EW, Dykstra DM, *et al.* Vascular access use in Europe and the United States: results from the DOPPS. *Kidney Int* 2002; 61: 305-16.
2. Rodriguez JA, Armadans L, Ferrer E, *et al.* The function of permanent vascular access. *Nephrol Dial Transplant* 2000; 15: 402-8.
3. Planken RN, Keuter HA, Hoeks APG, *et al.* Diameter measurements of the forearm cephalic vein prior to vascular access creation in end-stage renal disease patients: graduated pressure cuff versus tourniquet vessel dilatation. *Nephrol Dial Transplant* 2006; 21: 802-6.
4. Rooijens P, Burgmans J, Yo T, *et al.* Autogenous radial-cephalic or prosthetic brachial-antecubital forearm loop AVF in patients with compromised vessels? A randomized, multicenter study of the patency of primary hemodialysis access. *J Vasc Surg* 2005; 42: 481-6.
5. Van Hoek F, Scheltinga MR, Kouwenberg I, *et al.* Steal in hemodialysis patients depends on type of vascular access. *Eur J Vasc Endovasc Surg* 2006; 32: 710-7
6. Lin SL, Huang CH, Chen HS, *et al.* Effects of age and diabetes on blood flow rate and primary outcome of newly created hemodialysis arteriovenous fistulas. *Am J Nephrol* 1998; 18: 96-100.
7. Murphy GJ, White SA, Knight AJ, *et al.* Long-term results of arteriovenous fistulas using transposed autologous basilic vein. *Br J Surg* 2000; 87: 819-23.
8. Ruddle AC, Lear PA, Mitchell DC. The morbidity of secondary vascular access. A lifetime of intervention. *Eur J Vasc Endovasc Surg* 1999; 18: 30-4.
9. Yu VL, Goetz A, Wagner M, *et al. Staphylococcus aureus* nasal carriage and infection in patients on haemodialysis. *N Engl J Med* 1986; 315: 91-6.
10. Lemson MS, Tordoir JH, van Det RJ, *et al.* Effects of a venous cuff at the venous anastomosis of polytetrafluoroethylene grafts for hemodialysis vascular access. *J Vasc Surg* 2000; 32: 1155-63.
11. Sorom AJ, Hughes CB, McCarthy JT, *et al.* Prospective, randomized evaluation of a cuffed expanded polytetrafluoroethylene graft for haemodialysis vascular access. *Surgery* 2002; 132: 135-4.
12. NKF-DOQI clinical practice guidelines for vascular access. National Kidney Foundation - Dialysis Outcomes Quality Initiative. *Am J Kidney Dis* 1997; 30 (4, suppl 3).
13. Brady PS, Spence LD, Levitin A, *et al.* Efficacy of percutaneous fibrin sheath stripping in restoring patency of tunneled hemodialysis catheters. *Am J Roentgenol* 1999; 173: 1023-7.
14. Gray RJ, Levitin A, Buck D, *et al.* Percutaneous fibrin sheath stripping versus transcatheter urokinase infusion for malfunctioning well-positioned tunneled central venous dialysis catheters: a prospective, randomized trial. *J Vasc Interv Radiol* 2000; 11: 1121-9.
15. Merport M, Murphy TP, Egglin TK, *et al.* Fibrin sheath stripping versus catheter exchange for the treatment of failed tunneled hemodialysis catheters: randomized clinical trial. *J Vasc Interv Radiol* 2000; 11: 1115-20.

16. Henry ML. Routine surveillance in vascular access for hemodialysis. *Eur J Vasc Endovasc Surg* 2006; 32: 545-8.

17. Besarab A. Access monitoring is worthwhile and valuable. *Blood Purif* 2006; 24: 77-89.

18. Treacy PJ, Ragg JL, Snelling P, *et al.* Prediction of native arteriovenous fistulas using 'on-line' fistula flow measurements. *Nephrology* (Carlton) 2005; 10: 136-41.

19. Tessiotore N, Lipari G, Poli A, *et al.* Can blood flow surveillance and preemptive repair of subclinical stenosis prolong the useful life of arteriovenous fistulae? A randomized controlled study. *Nephrol Dial Transplant* 2004; 19: 2325-33.

20. Valentine RJ, Bouch CW, Scott DJ, *et al.* Do preoperative finger pressures predict early arterial steal in hemodialysis access patients? A prospective analysis. *J Vasc Surg* 2002; 36: 351-6.

21. Berman SS, Gentile AT, Glickman MH, *et al.* Distal revascularization-interval ligation for limb salvage and maintenance of dialysis access in ischemic steal syndrome. *J Vasc Surg* 1997; 26: 393-402.

22. Ehsan O, Bhattacharya D, Darwish A, *et al.* 'Extension technique': a modified technique for brachio-cephalic fistula to prevent dialysis access-associated steal syndrome. *Eur J Vasc Endovasc Surg* 2005; 29: 324-7.

Chapter 8
Biological and synthetic grafts for haemodialysis access

Janice Tsui MD MRCS, *Vascular Specialist Registrar*

George Hamilton MD FRCS, *Professor of Vascular Surgery*

Royal Free Hampstead NHS Trust

Royal Free & University College School of Medicine, London, UK

Introduction

Whilst the superiority of the autogenous arteriovenous (AV) fistula in terms of primary patency and lower complication rates is well recognised, autogenous conduits are not always available. In Europe, prosthetic material is used in 10-25% of all primary access procedures [1] and is often required in tertiary procedures. Material available for AV graft fistula construction includes prosthetic and biological grafts.

Properties of an ideal prosthetic graft

The ideal vascular graft should be thromboresistant, immunologically inert, resistant to infection, flexible yet strong, and inexpensive. In addition, grafts used for haemodialysis access should rapidly seal after puncture and be able to withstand repeated puncture trauma.

Unfortunately, none of the available grafts demonstrate all these properties and complications are common, resulting in significant morbidity.

Graft complications

Several studies have shown that the overall complication rates are higher for prosthetic AV grafts than for autogenous AV fistulae. In a study involving 1574 prosthetic grafts and 492 AV fistulae, prosthetic grafts had a 41% greater risk of primary failure, compared with AV fistulae and a 91% higher incidence of revision [2]. Specific complications are discussed below.

Thrombosis

Thrombosis is the commonest cause of access failure and prosthetic grafts have poorer patency than autogenous AVF [3]. Luminal thrombogenicity and anastomotic intimal hyperplasia are particular problems in prosthetic grafts and the latter result from vascular injury, loss of endothelial cells, compliance mismatch and altered haemodynamics.

Infection

Infection is more common in prosthetic grafts than in autogenous AV fistulae and is a devastating complication. In one prospective study, 8.2 infections/100 graft-years were found during a 4.5-year period. Early infection (within one month of graft placement) occurred in 15% of grafts and later infection (after one year of surgery) was found in 41% of grafts [4]. Gram-positive cocci, in particular *Staphylococcus aureus* and *Staphylococcus epidermidis*, are the commonest pathogens. Methicillin-resistant *S. aureus* (MRSA) is an increasing problem. Surgical removal of the infected graft is usually required. Biological grafts may be more resistant to infection.

Haemorrhage

Bleeding is more common in prosthetic grafts and may result from use of the graft prior to adequate incorporation into fibrous tissue, which may take 10 to 14 days, or from repeated needling of the same site. A self-sealing PTFE silicone graft designed for early cannulation unfortunately had higher rates of thrombosis [5].

Aneurysm formation

This occurs with both synthetic and biological grafts, and may result in thrombosis and rupture. Waiting a minimum period of three weeks after implantation of a biological AV graft before needling may reduce false aneurysm formation.

Steal

Distal ischaemia is more common in synthetic grafts compared to autogenous fistulae, but other factors are also important [6].

Biological grafts

Biological grafts have been used for many years but the only ones in current use are the saphenous and umbilical veins, and bovine ureter.

The main problems of biological grafts are biodegradation and immunogenicity, which are counteracted by cryopreservation and chemical treatment. Other problems include graft degeneration and aneurysm formation, particularly affecting arterial allografts. Cryopreserved venous allografts of the saphenous or femoral veins have been used for haemodialysis access with primary and secondary patency rates comparable to those of prosthetic AV grafts. In one centre, one-year primary graft patency rates of 49% and 65% were reported for cryopreserved femoral vein grafts and prosthetic AV grafts, respectively, and secondary patency rates for the two types of grafts were 75% and 78% [7]. Cryopreserved vein grafts were recommended initially for use in difficult situations such as in infected fields. A later study using cryopreserved femoral vein in AV grafts in patients at high risk of infection demonstrated high rates of graft infection (11 out of 20), with consequent graft rupture in six patients [8].

Human umbilical cord vein was first used by Dardik and early studies of its use in haemodialysis access showed poor overall patency, high rates of infection and aneurysmal degeneration [9]. It has since been used in a large number of patients for lower limb bypass procedures with reasonable patency rates, a low incidence of infection and no aneurysm formation [10]. Despite these results, it remains uncommonly used in haemodialysis access.

Early xenografts have also had disappointing results. The bovine carotid artery was first used in the 1970s. Although high overall patency rates have been reported, others have found poorer long-term patency with significant problems of degradation, aneurysm formation and infection rates of up to 25%.

More recently, a bovine mesenteric vein treated with glutaraldehyde crosslinking and gamma radiation (ProCol), has been used in the construction of AV grafts. Primary patency at 12 months was 35.6% compared to 28.4% for synthetic grafts and secondary patency at 24 months was 60.3% and 42.9% for the two groups, respectively. Complication rates including infection, dilation, and seroma formation were also lower for the bovine mesenteric vein grafts [11].

A modified bovine ureteric graft (SynerGraft) is also available with physical advantages of easy handling, a uniform diameter, optimal thickness, absence of valves and tributaries, and a high resistance to infection [12]. An early report suggests that bovine ureter seems to have similar one-year primary (29%) and secondary (81%) patencies to those reported for synthetic grafts with a low infection rate (5%) and only occasional aneurysm formation [13].

Synthetic grafts

Currently used synthetic graft material includes polytetrafluoroethylene (PTFE) and polyurethane.

Polytetrafluoroethylene

PTFE has been used in the expanded form (ePFTE) as a conduit for vascular access since the 1970s and remains the most commonly used graft material. However, it is not an ideal material: it is non-self-sealing, requiring prolonged compression after puncture, it is prone to false aneurysm formation, and is associated with high infection rates and suboptimal patency rates. In a systematic review, the primary patency rate for PTFE AV grafts was 58% at six months and 33% at 18 months; compared to corresponding figures of 72% and 51% for autogenous AV fistulae. Secondary patency rates for PTFE were also poorer at 76% at six months and 55% at 18 months, compared to rates of 86% and 77% for autogenous AV fistulae [3].

Modifications of the standard PTFE graft have been introduced in an attempt to improve results. Whilst wider grafts, an addition of a vein cuff or an expanded distal end (Venaflo) may improve patency rates, other modifications such as external supports and tapered ends have not been helpful.

Polyurethane

Polyurethane vascular access grafts were introduced in the 1990s and their advantages include easy cannulation, rapid compression haemostasis, early use post-implantation and reduced neointimal formation. However, they undergo hydrolytic degradation leading to aneurysm formation. Newer polyurethanes have been manufactured to combat this problem. These newer grafts may have advantages over ePTFE in terms of haemostasis and reduced aneursymal dilatation, but no advantage in patency rates have been shown with one-year cumulative patency rates of 53% for polyurethane and 71% for ePTFE grafts [14].

A summary of graft materials and their respective patencies is presented in Table 1.

Future grafts

Different techniques are under development to manufacture grafts which match the autogenous conduit more closely and to overcome some of the above problems.

Table 1 Summary of graft materials for haemodialysis access.

Graft material	Primary patency	Secondary patency	Problems
Autogenous AVF	72% at 6 months, 51% at 18 months [3]	85% at 6 months, 77% at 18 months [3]	Unavailable in up to 25% procedures
Saphenous/ femoral veins	49% at 1 year [7]	75% at 1 year [7]	Infection, rupture
Human umbilical cord	24% [9]	84% [9]	Infection, aneurysm formation
Bovine mesenteric vein (ProCol)	36% at 1 year [11]	60% at 2 years [11]	Needs more data
Bovine ureteric graft (SynerGraft)	29% at 1 year [13]	81% at 1 year [13]	Needs more data
ePTFE	58% at 6 months, 33% at 18 months [3]	71% cumulative at 1 year [14]	Non-self-sealing, infection, aneurysm formation
Polyurethane	-	53% cumulative at 1 year [14]	Needs more data

Evidence from large randomised controlled trials is generally lacking and different controls have been used in case-controlled studies. The systematic review on PTFE AV grafts compared patency rates with those of autogenous AV fistulae [3], whilst results of biological grafts are compared to those of prosthetic grafts [11, 13] and polyurethane compared to ePTFE grafts [14].

Endothelial cell seeding

The endothelium plays a vital role in the patency of native blood vessels and the aim of endothelial cell seeding is to line the luminal surface of prosthetic grafts with a confluent endothelial monolayer. Studies have shown that endothelial seeded grafts have normal endothelial cell activity, are less thrombogenic and have better patency rates. These grafts have also been shown in animal models to have higher resistance to bacterial infection. Endothelial seeded ePTFE grafts have been used in infra-inguinal reconstructions with a 65% patency rate at nine years in 100 patients [15], and in coronary artery bypass surgery, a 90.5% patency rate at 28 months has been reported [16].

Tissue-engineered autogenous grafts

Several groups have been working on producing a totally autogenous tissue-engineered graft. L'Heureux wrapped sheets of cultured smooth muscle cells around a tubular support to produce a media, with an adventitia composed of an outer sheet of cultured fibroblasts. A confluent layer of endothelial cells was then seeded onto the luminal surface after removal of the tubular support. The resulting graft was able to withstand physiological pressures, with both the endothelial cells and the smooth muscle cells showing normal functional characteristics [17]. Further developments in this field are rapidly progressing and show potential for clinical application in the near future.

Polyurethane grafts

Biostable polyurethane polymers have been recently developed, with one graft for renal access achieving CE marking and transiently introduced to the European market (Expedial, Le Maitre, Inc). This graft was compliant and had excellent puncture sealing due to its sponge-like wall structure, but unfortunately had a thrombogenic surface resulting in a high failure rate at implantation and on compression. This graft is no longer in production but further access grafts made of novel biostable polyurethane polymers which are non-thrombogenic are currently under development;

these grafts will have similar compliance, puncture-sealing properties and promise to have a low risk of thrombosis [18].

Conclusions

The main advantages of synthetic grafts are availability, ease of handling and suitability for earlier use. However, currently available materials are associated with poor patency rates, high infection risk and aneurysm formation. Biological grafts theoretically have a higher resistance to infection compared to synthetic grafts but are also prone to degeneration and aneurysm formation.

In a significant proportion of patients requiring dialysis, an AV graft fistula using these materials may be the only option available. Careful access planning with pre-operative imaging, meticulous surgical technique, postoperative graft surveillance, and early endovascular and surgical intervention contribute to better results [19] and can be adopted by all units.

Newer materials using tissue-engineering technology may be available in the near future with the potential to produce results similar to those of the autogenous AV fistula.

Key Summary

◆ An autogenous AV fistula is the primary vascular access of choice in most patients.

◆ The commonest synthetic graft currently used is expanded PTFE. Polyurethane has not shown clear clinical advantages.

◆ Biological graft materials currently available are the allogenic saphenous and umbilical veins. Bovine mesenteric vein and bovine ureteric graft may be new alternatives.

◆ Common complications included thrombosis, infection, and aneurysm formation.

◆ Tissue-engineered and novel polyurethane grafts may be available in the future.

References

1. Allon M, Robbin ML. Increasing arteriovenous fistulas in hemodialysis patients: problems and solutions. *Kidney Int* 2002; 62: 1109-24.
2. Gibson KD, Gillen DL, Caps MT, *et al.* Vascular access survival and incidence of revisions: a comparison of prosthetic grafts, simple autogenous fistulas, and venous transposition fistulas from the United States Renal Data System Dialysis Morbidity and Mortality Study. *J Vasc Surg* 2001; 34: 694-700.
3. Huber TS, Carter JW, Carter RL, *et al.* Patency of autogenous and polytetrafluoroethylene upper extremity arteriovenous hemodialysis accesses: a systematic review. *J Vasc Surg* 2003; 38: 1005-11.
4. Minga TE, Flanagan KH, Allon M. Clinical consequences of infected arteriovenous grafts in hemodialysis patients. *Am J Kidney Dis* 2001; 38: 975-8.
5. Coyne DW, Lowell JA, Windus DW, *et al.* Comparison of survival of an expanded polytetrafluoroethylene graft designed for early cannulation to standard wall polytetrafluoroethylene grafts. *J Am Coll Surg* 1996; 183: 401-5.

6.   Davidson D, Louridas G, Guzman R, *et al*. Steal syndrome complicating upper extremity hemoaccess procedures: incidence and risk factors. *Can J Surg* 2003; 46: 408-12.

7.   Matsuura JH, Johansen KH, Rosenthal D, *et al*. Cryopreserved femoral vein grafts for difficult hemodialysis access. *Ann Vasc Surg* 2000; 14: 50-5.

8.   Bolton WD, Cull DL, Taylor SM, *et al*. The use of cryopreserved femoral vein grafts for hemodialysis access in patients at high risk for infection: a word of caution. *J Vasc Surg* 2002; 36: 464-8.

9.   Jorgensen L, Bilde T, Kvist KJ, *et al*. Human umbilical vein for vascular access in chronic hemodialysis. *Scand J Urol Nephrol* 1985; 19: 49-53.

10.   Dardik H, Wengerter K, Qin F, *et al*. Comparative decades of experience with glutaraldehyde-tanned human umbilical cord vein graft for lower limb revascularization: an analysis of 1275 cases. *J Vasc Surg* 2002; 35: 64-71.

11.   Katzman HE, Glickman MH, Schild AF, *et al*. Multicenter evaluation of the bovine mesenteric vein bioprostheses for hemodialysis access in patients with an earlier failed prosthetic graft. *J Am Coll Surg* 2005; 201: 223-30.

12.   Matsuura JH, Black KS, Levitt AB, *et al*. Cellular remodeling of depopulated bovine ureter used as an arteriovenous graft in the canine model. *J Am Coll Surg* 2004; 198: 778-83.

13.   Darby CR, Roy D, Deardon D, *et al*. Depopulated bovine ureteric xenograft for complex haemodialysis vascular access. *Eur J Vasc Endovasc Surg* 2006; 31: 181-6.

14.   Nakagawa Y, Ota K, Sato Y, *et al*. Clinical trial of new polyurethane vascular grafts for hemodialysis: compared with expanded polytetrafluoroethylene grafts. *Artif Organs* 1995; 19: 1227-32.

15.   Deutsch M, Meinhart J, Fischlein T, *et al*. Clinical autologous *in vitro* endothelialization of infrainguinal ePTFE grafts in 100 patients: a 9-year experience. *Surgery* 1999; 126: 847-55.

16.   Laube HR, Duwe J, Rutsch W, *et al*. Clinical experience with autologous endothelial cell-seeded polytetrafluoroethylene coronary artery bypass grafts. *J Thorac Cardiovasc Surg* 2000; 120: 134-41.

17.   L'Heureux N, Dusserre N, Konig G, *et al*. Human tissue-engineered blood vessels for adult arterial revascularization. *Nat Med* 2006; 12: 361-5.

18.   Kannan RY, Salacinski HJ, Edirisinghe MJ, *et al*. Polyhedral oligomeric silsequioxane-polyurethane nanocomposite microvessels for an artificial capillary bed. *Biomaterials* 2006; 27: 4618-26.

19.   Shemesh D, Olsha O, Berelowitz D, *et al*. Integrated approach to construction and maintenance of prosthetic arteriovenous access for hemodialysis. *Vascular* 2004; 12: 243-55.

Chapter 9

Complex vascular access

Nung Rudarakanchana PhD MRCS

Senior House Officer, Charing Cross Hospital, London, UK

Alun H Davies MA DM FRCS

Reader in Surgery and Consultant Surgeon, Imperial College School of Medicine,

Charing Cross Hospital, London, UK

Introduction

The incidence of end-stage renal failure in the UK is currently estimated at 500 per million. With improving medical treatment and increasing life expectancy, the dialysis-dependent population in this country is set to significantly increase over the coming years. The provision of this growing population with safe, effective and durable vascular access is a major challenge for the modern surgeon.

Dialysis Outcomes Quality Initiative clinical practice guidelines published in 2006 by the National Kidney Foundation (USA) offer a structured approach to vascular access formation. These guidelines are based on current evidence and recommend distal upper limb native arteriovenous (AV) fistulae (radiocephalic) in preference to proximal native fistulae (brachiocephalic, basilic vein transposition) and over prosthetic graft placement (forearm loop, upper-arm straight, curve or loop). Furthermore, these guidelines advise that all upper extremity options should be exhausted before resorting to vascular access in the thigh because of the high risk of infection.

In current practice it is increasingly common to encounter patients in whom all these standard options for dialysis access have been exhausted. One study suggests that 38% of patients undergoing dialysis through temporary catheters and 27% through permanent catheters will present with central venous stenosis or obstruction [1]. Consequential limitation of fistula flow and symptomatic facial or limb oedema are familiar problems.

The additional problems of inadequate peripheral vein, inadequate arterial inflow secondary to arterial disease and obesity in this patient population are also rising. These patients require the formation of complex (exotic, extra-anatomic) vascular access. This chapter reviews the literature on central and lower limb AV fistulae and novel arterio-arterial loop fistulae.

Assessment for complex vascular access

The assessment of patients for the formation of complex vascular access follows that of the standard approach to all patients requiring permanent haemodialysis access: access history, including limb oedema and central vein cannulation, physical examination and non-invasive vascular imaging to define both arterial and venous systems. In addition, formal delineation of the central venous system and angiography or magnetic resonance angiography may be required to confirm the optimal choice of access.

Anterior chest wall arteriovenous graft fistulae

First advocated by Manning in 1975, anterior chest wall graft fistulae include grafts based on the axillary or subclavian arteries with outflow through either axillary or jugular veins [2]. These bypasses are advocated in patients in whom all upper limb access options have been exhausted, either due to thrombosis or inadequate vessel calibre, and who have a patent superior vena cava or in patients with unilateral subclavian artery or vein occlusion. Steal syndrome following grafts based on the axillary artery is a rare occurrence, due to the abundant collateral flow surrounding the vessel, and thus these procedures are suitable options in patients who are at high risk of this complication.

Axillo-axillary ('necklace') and axillojugular bypass graft fistulae (Figure 1)

The first necklace (axillo-axillary) bypass was reported in 1978 by Garcia-Rinaldi and von Koch [3]. Bilateral infraclavicular incisions are made and the axillary vessels are exposed medial to the insertion of the

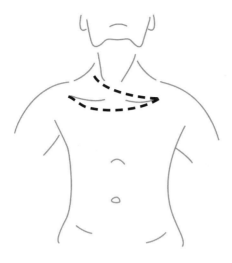

Figure 1 Axillo-axillary and axillojugular graft fistulae.

pectoralis minor muscle. A prosthetic graft is tunnelled in the subdermal plane over the superior third of the sternum and cephalad to any breast tissue. The graft is anastomosed from an axillary artery to the contralateral axillary vein.

Axillojugular bypass is a suitable alternative configuration in patients with subclavian vein stenosis. The jugular vein is exposed via a supraclavicular incision over the sternocleidomastoid muscle and the graft is tunnelled over the clavicle from an axillary artery to the contralateral internal jugular vein.

The use of axillo-axillary and axillojugular loop bypass, in which the graft is anastomosed from an axillary artery to the ipsilateral axillary or internal jugular vein, has been reported in cases of unilateral central vein stenosis [4]. The relative merits of straight versus loop grafts continue to be debated in present literature: the loop configuration is thought to dissipate high arterial pressure more evenly throughout the graft; the straight configuration may decrease the risk of graft kinking with subsequent occlusion and thrombosis.

The largest published series of axillo-axillary and axillojugular bypass grafts reported a 77% three-year cumulative patency rate in over 50 patients [5]. A standard-walled 6mm polytetrafluoroethylene (PTFE) graft was used. There were no cases of postoperative steal syndrome. Thrombosis was the major cause of graft loss; this was treated by thrombectomy with or without revision of the venous anastomosis. In a more recent study involving 26 patients, one-year primary and secondary graft patency rates were 33% and 57%, respectively [4]. Heparin-coated polycarbonate/urethane grafts, which are self-sealing and allow early vascular access, and extended PTFE grafts were used. Early complications of facial oedema and contralateral hemiparesis were reported; in both cases these symptoms spontaneously resolved. Late complications included seroma, pseudoaneurysm and graft infection.

In cases where there is no suitable axillary or internal jugular vein target, alternate venous outflow conduits may be considered.

Axillo-iliac bypass graft fistulae (Figure 2)

Axillo-iliac bypass is undertaken via an infraclavicular incision to expose the axillary artery and an extraperitoneal approach to expose the ipsilateral iliac vein. The graft is tunnelled subcutaneously along the anterior axillary line and anastomosed.

A series of nine axillo-iliac graft fistulae in eight patients using an externally-splinted PTFE graft tunnelled beneath the pectoralis major muscle was reported [6]. Two patients died with functioning grafts and six out of eight patients had functioning grafts at one year. There were no postoperative episodes of thrombosis or infection at one-year follow-up. Two patients developed lower limb oedema secondary to proximal iliac vein stricture and retrograde flow through the femoral vein. This venous hypertension was successfully decompressed in both patients by femoral-femoral venous bypass.

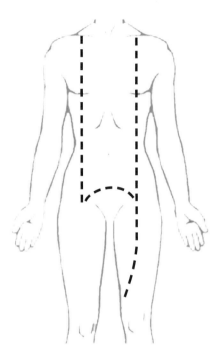

Figure 2 Axillo-iliac, axillopopliteal and femorofemoral graft fistulae.

In more recent literature, a study of five axillo-iliac graft fistulae was published [7]. This group utilised a non-externally supported 7mm PTFE graft tunnelled subcutaneously. The primary patency rate was 80% at six months and four out of five patients had usable grafts at one year. Postoperatively, there were no cases of steal syndrome and no significant discrepancy between arm pressures. Two episodes of graft occlusion occurred; in both cases flow was successfully restored by thrombectomy. One patient developed postoperative lower limb swelling; this resolved with conservative management.

Axillofemoral bypass graft fistulae

There are only two reports of axillary artery to common femoral vein graft fistulae in the literature [8, 9]: one group reported two adult cases of axillofemoral bypass with satisfactory results, and a second reported an axillofemoral graft in a child as part of a study of haemodialysis access in the paediatric patient population.

Axillopopliteal bypass graft fistulae (Figure 2)

Some authors advocate the use of the axillary artery to popliteal vein graft in patients with central venous obstruction in whom all upper limb vascular access options have been exhausted and who are not suitable for lower limb fistulae because of peripheral vascular disease [10]. The technique described by this group utilises an infraclavicular approach to the second part of the axillary artery and a thigh incision over the subsartorial canal to expose the superficial femoral/popliteal vein. An 8mm reinforced PTFE graft is tunnelled subcutaneously in two stages along the anterior axillary line: initially from the subclavian position to a separate skin incision in the flank and then further over the abdomen and onto the anterolateral aspect of the thigh. All reinforcing rings, except for those in the lower abdominal-inguinal section of the graft, are removed to enable cannulation.

The initial case study describing this technique reported postoperative seroma and lower limb swelling, due to common iliac vein stenosis, in one patient and no postoperative complications in the other [10]. Both grafts allowed initial satisfactory dialysis flows. The same group further reported a series of five axillopopliteal graft fistulae as part of a larger study in 2006 [11]. Four out of the five patients had usable grafts at the end of the study (median follow-up 22 months, range 2-30 months). The remaining patient suffered rapid onset of severe steal syndrome which necessitated tying off of the fistula at three weeks postoperatively. This group suggests a decreased risk of infection as a result of contamination from the groin during surgery or from cannulation, as an advantage of axillopopliteal over axillofemoral grafts. In addition, longer bypasses allow easier rotation of cannulation sites. However, theoretical disadvantages of the axillopopliteal configuration include an increased risk of graft kinking and possible decreased flow rates due to the peripheral venous outflow.

Axillorenal bypass graft fistulae

There has been a single case report of axillorenal graft fistulae in a patient with supra-superior vena caval and infrarenal pan-venous occlusion [12]. The technique described in this case employs a standard infraclavicular incision to expose the axillary artery and a left subcostal incision to allow a retroperitoneal approach to the renal vein. A Vectra (Thoratec) graft is tunnelled subcutaneously from the axillary artery lateral to the nipple and brought below the eleventh rib. Both arterial and venous ends are anastomosed end-to-side. Although initial dialysis flow was satisfactory, the fistula required two revisions: initially with an interposition graft to correct excessive angulation at the costal margin and then rectification of a twisted venous anastomosis. One thrombectomy and two percutaneous venoplasty procedures were required to maintain adequate dialysis flow. However, the graft remained usable at 18 months postoperatively. The report posits several advantages of this fistula configuration, including the proximity of the venous anastomosis to the inferior vena cava resulting in a low resistance to flow and therefore possibly improved graft patency, and the low likelihood of prior renal vein cannulation. The authors do acknowledge that the placing of the graft does require improvement in order to decrease the risk of kinking and thrombosis.

Groin and lower limb arteriovenous graft fistulae

Historically, the insertion of a lower limb prosthetic graft for vascular access was deemed unacceptable; use of the Thomas shunt, an externalised AV fistula comprising a velour-covered tube cemented to a fabric patch, led to high rates of infection, thrombosis and bleeding. A seminal paper by Morgan *et al* in 1980 [13] reported a nine-year retrospective study on 161 patients with femoral triangle vascular access. Grafts used included the Thomas shunt, saphenous vein, bovine vessel, Sparks mandril and PTFE. Twenty-seven femoral triangle infections (17%) were reported with a subsequent amputation rate of 22% and mortality rate of 18% in these patients. A more recent retrospective five-year study involving 39 patients with femoral arteriovenous dialysis grafts reported postoperative graft infection in 18% of patients, severe leg ischaemia in 16% and lower limb amputation in 7%. Graft patency was 47% at two-year follow-up [14]. The debate as to whether the placement of femoral triangle graft fistulae is an acceptable practice is on-going, although undoubtedly there exists a population of patients in which this is the only remaining option for vascular access. Most surgeons consider significant peripheral vascular disease as a contraindication to femoral arteriovenous graft fistulae.

Lower limb native arteriovenous fistulae

Overall, native AV fistulae have lower rates of thrombosis and infection and increased survival rates, as compared to graft fistulae. Therefore, in patients with no remaining upper limb access options, native lower limb fistulae should initially be considered.

Superficial femoral vein transposition

Transposition of the superficial femoral vein is undertaken via a thigh incision over the subsartorial canal. The adductor magnus tendon is divided and the vein is mobilised from the popliteal fossa to the junction of the vein with the profunda femoral vein. The vein is transposed superficially and anastomosed end-to-side to the distal superficial femoral artery between the divided adductor magnus tendon and the inferior border of sartorius muscle.

A retrospective study involving 25 patients undergoing superficial vein transposition, reported primary and secondary patency rates of 73% and 86% at one year [15]. Although no fistula infections were recorded, there were major wound complications in seven patients, steal syndrome requiring further intervention in eight patients and acute compartment syndrome necessitating amputation in one patient. More recently, the same group have examined strategies to reduce the incidence of ischaemic complications. In a study of 46 patients, superficial femoral vein tapering was found to significantly reduce the risk of postoperative steal syndrome; this modification to the procedure did not affect patency rates. Superficial femoral vein transposition and femoral loop grafts were compared in a prospective trial of 30 patients [16]. The incidence of steal syndrome and infection rates were not significantly different between the two groups. However, among the six infections in patients undergoing femoral loop grafts, four required removal of the prosthesis, whereas only one fistula was closed in the superficial femoral vein transposition group. One-year patency rates were significantly better in patients undergoing superficial vein transposition (87% versus 38%).

Saphenous vein fistulae

Fistulae based on the saphenous vein include saphenous vein/popliteal artery fistula, saphenous vein loop/femoral artery fistula, and saphenous vein transposition. However, fistula patency rates are often disappointing and many additional procedures, such as surgical revision and dilatation, are frequently required. Vein calibre, positioning of vein and patient body habitus are all important factors in the success or otherwise of these fistulae.

Femorofemoral ('bikini') bypass graft fistulae (Figure 2)

The formation of a femorofemoral (bikini) graft fistula in a patient with severe upper limb arterial disease and steal syndrome resulting from a previous brachiocephalic fistula has been described [11]. This patient refused a necklace bypass or thigh fistula because of cosmetic reasons. The technique employed in this case utilises bilateral groin incisions to expose the common femoral vessels. The graft is tunnelled subcutaneously on the anterior aspect of the lower abdominal wall below the umbilicus. The graft is anastomosed end-to-side with a common femoral artery and the contralateral common femoral vein. In this patient a 6mm externally supported PTFE graft was used. The graft remained in use at the end of the study (median follow-up 22 months, range 2-30 months).

Femorofemoral loop graft fistulae have been used by certain groups since the 1980s. The femoral vessels are exposed via a groin incision and the graft is tunnelled subcutaneously so that the distal end of the loop lies approximately 8-10cm above the knee. A distal incision at this level is made to ensure that the graft lies flat without kinking. The average length of the loop is approximately 25-30cm. The graft is anastomosed end-to-side with the superficial femoral artery and the ipsilateral femoral vein.

A 14-year retrospective study reported a series of 35 patients and 37 femorofemoral loop 6mm PTFE grafts [17]. There were three cases of immediate graft thrombosis. Late postoperative complications included distal ischaemia with worsening claudication in four patients and necessitating a foot amputation in one diabetic patient, graft thrombosis in four patients and Gram-negative graft infections in two patients. Graft patency was 73% at one year and 33% at three years, comparable with upper limb grafts, and efficiency of haemodialysis was adequate. A second study involving 46 patients and 49 femorofemoral loop grafts reported graft patency at 85% at one year and 70% at three years. However, postoperative complication rates were significant with graft thrombosis and infection occurring in 52% and 35% of patients, respectively.

More recently, a group have advocated the use of a mid-thigh loop graft fistula based off the superficial femoral artery and vein [18]. They reported a series of 46 such grafts in 38 patients over a three-year period and found primary and secondary graft patency rates of 40% and 68% at one year and 18% and 43% at two years, respectively. There were ten graft infections (21%) necessitating graft removal. The authors highlighted the advantage of the mid-thigh loop graft in preserving the proximal vasculature and therefore permitting graft revision or subsequent proximal graft replacement.

Femoral artery to right atrium bypass graft fistulae

In an interesting case, Chemla *et al* [11] reported the formation of a unique graft fistula from the superficial femoral artery to the superior vena cava in a patient with superior and inferior vena cava thrombosis. In this technique the right atrium and great vessels are exposed via a median sternotomy (cardiopulmonary bypass is not necessary) and the femoral vessels are dissected through a groin incision. The graft is tunnelled subcutaneously along the lateral aspect of the abdomen and chest wall. A further incision is made on the lateral chest wall and the graft is inserted into the thorax through the second intercostal space. The graft is anastomosed end-to-side with the superficial femoral artery and the superior vena cava above the right atrium and below the azygos vein. A 6mm externally supported

PTFE graft was used in this case. Although this patient required intensive care support postoperatively, the graft remained in use at the end of the study (median follow-up 22 months, range 2-30 months).

Arterio-arterial loop graft fistulae

The use of an artery as permanent vascular access for haemodialysis was first published in 1969 by Brittinger *et al* [19], utilising a subcutaneously fixed superficial femoral artery. A series of seven patients with arterial femoropopliteal jump grafts reported satisfactory results; bovine carotid artery was used as a graft [20]. More recently, two separate groups have produced studies on arterio-arterial loop graft fistulae. Indications for such grafts include occlusion of central veins, severe steal syndrome and, rarely, high output cardiac failure. Axillary loop graft fistulae are performed via a standard infraclavicular incision to expose the axillary artery and the graft is placed in a loop configuration subcutaneously in the anterior chest wall. The axillary artery is occluded and the graft is interpositioned and anastomosed end-to-end with the artery. A similar procedure is used to create femoral loop graft fistulae centred on the common femoral artery.

In the largest published study of arterio-arterial graft fistulae, 34 patients received 36 loop graft fistulae as vascular access (31 axillary loops and five femoral loops) [21]. Grafts were 6 or 7mm PTFE. Primary patency was 73% and 54% and secondary patency was 96% and 87% at one year and three years, respectively. There were no early postoperative complications. Graft thrombosis occurred during the late postoperative period in 15 patients (42%); in these situations the femoral loops required immediate thrombectomy, whereas occlusion of the axillary loops caused only mild distal ischaemia. Four loop grafts were abandoned due to repeated thromboses or anastomotic stenosis; in two cases a new loop fistula was formed, in the remaining two cases femoral arteriovenous grafts were created. Six grafts developed pseudoaneurysms following puncture, necessitating graft reconstructions. Painful reperfusion of the distal arteries was observed in a few cases of high-flow dialysis. Flow rates sufficient for haemodialysis were achieved by all but two loop grafts. A contemporary study of 20 patients with axillary loop fistulae reported primary and secondary patency rates of 90% and 93%, respectively.

The advantages of arterio-arterial loop grafts over arteriovenous grafts are three-fold: target venous outflow is not required; distal perfusion is not decreased, negating the potential for steal syndrome; and cardiac load is not increased. An intervention rate of 0.47 procedures per patient per year was recorded in one study [21], comparable with the rates for arteriovenous grafts. However, potential problems of arterio-arterial loop grafts include: occlusion of the graft with consequent distal ischaemia; graft infection requiring graft removal and arterial reconstruction; distal embolisation; pseudoaneurysm formation; and painful reperfusion on dialysis through the fistula.

Conclusions

The increasing numbers of patients who require the formation of complex vascular access represent a significant challenge to the modern surgeon. Anterior chest wall AV fistulae (axillo-axillary, axillojugular, axillo-iliac, axillofemoral and axillopopliteal), lower limb native AV fistulae (superficial femoral vein transposition, saphenous vein fistulae), and groin arteriovenous graft fistulae (femorofemoral) have been utilised with success in patients who have exhausted all conventional forms of vascular access. More creative graft fistulae, such as axillorenal and femoro-atrial arteriovenous grafts, and axillo-axillary and femorofemoral arterio-arterial grafts, are being developed as individual patient cases dictate. Postoperative complications of thrombosis, infection and distal ischaemia are significant and must be taken in context of this high-risk patient population.

Key Summary

◆ The need for complex (exotic, extra-anatomic) vascular access is increasing. In addition to failure of primary and secondary vascular access, the problems of central vein stenosis, inadequate peripheral vein, inadequate arterial inflow secondary to arterial disease and obesity must be considered.

◆ Anterior chest wall graft fistulae based off the axillary artery include axillo-axillary (necklace), axillojugular, axillo-iliac, axillofemoral and axillopopliteal arteriovenous grafts. These are particularly useful in patients who are at high risk of developing steal syndrome. Axillorenal and femoro-atrial graft fistulae have been reported in unique cases.

◆ Reported rates of infection and distal ischaemia with femoral arteriovenous grafts vary. Peripheral vascular disease is a contraindication to femoral graft fistula.

◆ Lower limb native fistulae include superficial vein transposition and saphenous vein fistulae. Loop and crossover femorofemoral arteriovenous graft fistulae have been reported.

◆ Arterio-arterial axillary and femoral loop graft fistulae are novel further options.

References

1. Surratt RS, Picus D, Hicks ME, *et al*. The importance of pre-operative evaluation of the subclavian vein in dialysis access planning. *AJR Am J Roentgenol* 1991; 156(3): 623-5.
2. Manning LG, Mozersky DJ, Murray HM, Hagood CO. Axillary-axillary bovine arteriovenous fistula for hemodialysis. *Arch Surg* 1975; 110(1): 114-5.

3. Garcia-Rinaldi R, von Koch L. The axillary artery to axillary vein bovine graft for circulatory access: surgical considerations. *Am J Surg* 1978; 135(2): 265-8.

4. Hazinedaroglu S, Karakayali F, Tuzuner A, *et al*. Exotic arteriovenous fistulas for hemodialysis. *Transplant Proc* 2004; 36(1): 59-64.

5. McCann RL. Vascular access for the 'difficult' patient. In: Conlon PJ, Schwab SJ, Nicholson M, Eds. *Hemodialysis Vascular Access, Practice and Problems*. Oxford University Press: Oxford, 2001.

6. Cimochowski GE, Harter HR, Rutherford WE, *et al*. Axillary artery to iliac vein vascular access using an externally supported prosthetic graft. A new procedure for the recalcitrant secondary access patient. *ASAIO Trans* 1987; 33(3): 123-8.

7. Hamish M, Shalhoub J, Rodd CD, Davies AH. Axillo-iliac conduit for haemodialysis vascular access. *Eur J Vasc Endovasc Surg* 2006; 31(5): 530-4.

8. Rueckmann I, Berry C, Ouriel K, Hoffart N. The synthetic axillofemoral graft for hemodialysis access. *Anna J* 1991; 18(6): 567-71.

9. Lumsden AB, MacDonald MJ, Allen RC, Dodson TF. Hemodialysis access in the pediatric patient population. *Am J Surg* 1994; 168(2): 197-201.

10. Calder FR, Chemla ES, Anderson L, Chang RW. The axillary artery-popliteal vein extended polytetrafluoroethylene graft: a new technique for the complicated dialysis access patient. *Nephrol Dial Transplant* 2004; 19(4): 998-1000.

11. Chemla ES, Morsy M, Anderson L, Makanjuola D. Complex bypasses and fistulas for difficult hemodialysis access: a prospective, single-center experience. *Semin Dial* 2006; 19(3): 246-50.

12. Karp SJ, Hawxby A, Burdick JF. Axillorenal arteriovenous graft: a new approach for dialysis access. *J Vasc Surg* 2004; 40(2): 379-80.

13. Morgan AP, Knight DC, Tilney NL, Lazarus JM. Femoral triangle sepsis in dialysis patients: frequency, management, and outcome. *Ann Surg* 1980; 191(4): 460-4.

14. Taylor SM, Eaves GL, Weatherford DA, *et al*. Results and complications of arteriovenous access dialysis grafts in the lower extremity: a five year review. *Am Surg* 1996; 62(3): 188-91.

15. Gradman WS, Cohen W, Haji-Aghaii M. Arteriovenous fistula construction in the thigh with transposed superficial femoral vein: our initial experience. *J Vasc Surg* 2001; 33(5): 968-75.

16. Hazinedaroglu SM, Tuzuner A, Ayli D, *et al*. Femoral vein transposition versus femoral loop grafts for hemodialysis: a prospective evaluation. *Transplant Proc* 2004; 36(1): 65-7.

17. Korzets A, Ori Y, Baytner S, *et al*. The femoral artery-femoral vein polytetrafluoroethylene graft: a 14-year retrospective study. *Nephrol Dial Transplant* 1998; 13(5): 1215-20.

18. Scott JD, Cull DL, Kalbaugh CA, *et al*. The mid-thigh loop arteriovenous graft: patient selection, technique, and results. *Am Surg* 2006; 72(9): 825-8.

19. Brittinger WD, Strauch M, Huber W, *et al*. Shuntless hemodialysis by means of puncture of the subcutaneously fixed superficial femoral artery. First dialysis experiences. *Klin Wochenschr* 1969; 47(15): 824-6.

20. Butt KM, Kountz SL. A new vascular access for hemodialysis: the arterial jump graft. *Surgery* 1976; 79(4): 476-9.

21. Zanow J, Kruger U, Petzold M, *et al*. Arterioarterial prosthetic loop: a new approach for hemodialysis access. *J Vasc Surg* 2005; 41(6): 1007-12.

Chapter 10
Complications of access surgery

Ali Bakran FRCS (Eng) FRCS (Edin), *Consultant Vascular & Transplant Surgeon*
Royal Liverpool University Hospital, Liverpool, UK

Introduction

Vascular access is crucial to the well-being of the haemodialysis patient. Access malfunction or occlusion has serious consequences, often requiring temporary haemodialysis through a central venous dialysis catheter, which increases morbidity and mortality [1]. Consideration of access complications must therefore take into account not only those of the access itself but also the resultant risks of the temporary access.

Early complications

Haemorrhage

Haemorrhage can manifest as peri-anastomotic haematoma or frank bleeding. The bleeding most often occurs from the anastomosis but may also result from side branch ligature slippage. It is more likely to occur if intravenous heparin has been given and reversal of anticoagulation with protamine sulphate may be appropriate if bleeding is persistent and extensive. The site of haemorrhage is usually easy to detect and external compression simply applied. If the bleeding is self-limiting and the haematoma small, then no further procedure need be performed. However, a haematoma may compress the anastomosis, prevent dilatation of the vein, and cause fistula thrombosis or infection, particularly if a prosthetic graft is used. Occasionally even wound dehiscence may occur. Therefore, exploration and evacuation of a significant haematoma is advisable. Clearly, haemorrhage that persists despite compression requires re-exploration and under-running of the bleeding point.

Wound infection

Autogenous fistula wounds, whether at the wrist, antecubital fossa, axilla or thigh, infrequently become infected but usually respond to systemic antibiotic therapy. Infection of a wound overlying a prosthetic arteriovenous (AV) fistula has potentially serious consequences with risk of graft infection. In view of the known reduced immune function in patients with renal failure, and despite the clean anastomosis between graft and vessels, it is advisable to give systemic antibiotic prophylaxis at the time of anaesthetic induction to cover the procedure, particularly against *Staphylococcus aureus* infection. Any discharge from such wounds should be sent for microbiological culture and anti-staphylococcal therapy, such as flucloxacillin, should be commenced, whilst awaiting confirmation of the organism and antibiotic sensitivity [2]. If frank pus emanates from such a wound then re-exploration and removal of the prosthetic graft is mandatory. Secondary haemorrhage from such a wound can be catastrophic.

Sometimes there is redness along the line of the graft tunnel, which may be a direct response to the tunnelling procedure and may settle with anti-inflammatory agents. Occasionally such wounds progress to tunnel infection, in which case the graft should be removed.

Thrombosis

Thrombosis of an AV fistula can occur soon after completion of the anastomosis, in the recovery suite, on return to the ward or within a few weeks after surgery. Intra or peri-operative thrombosis may be due to technical factors, poor selection of small or diseased vessels, or, less frequently, a generalised thrombotic tendency. If the fistula, artery and vein are of reasonable calibre then urgent re-exploration is appropriate and should be followed by postoperative heparinisation for 24 hours. The vein may be twisted or the arterial inflow to the fistula kinked, in which case local revision may be all that is needed. However, the other option is to redo the fistula at a slightly more proximal site. General anaesthesia usually results in a fall in blood pressure and if this occurs, it is advisable to ask the anaesthetist to raise the blood pressure above 100mmHg systolic before establishing flow (especially through a prosthetic graft) and use systemic heparinisation to prevent thrombosis. If the cause of thrombosis remains unclear on re-exploration, then systemic heparinisation for at least 24 hours is warranted. Grafts frequently thrombose with a blood pressure less than 100mmHg, so they should be avoided in patients who consistently run a low blood pressure, especially if they become haemodynamically unstable during dialysis.

Frequently, a radiocephalic AV fistula is performed with no investigation other than examination of the distended cephalic vein with a proximal tourniquet. However, pre-operative duplex scanning has been shown to be useful for the pre-selection of vessels prior to AV fistula creation [3, 4]. Several studies have shown that a minimum arterial and venous diameter is necessary for a successful outcome. The radial artery may be small, particularly in women, or significantly diseased in the diabetic. For graft fistulae, a small outflow vein may lead to early thrombosis. The venous diameter should therefore be at least 3mm and the US DOQI guidelines suggest a minimum diameter as high as 4mm for grafts (see Chapter 5) [5]. Since prosthetic grafts should only be placed when all possible autogenous fistula options have been utilised, including the brachiobasilic AV fistula, the brachio-axillary graft would satisfy this requirement.

Failure of maturation

In contrast to graft fistulae, which can usually be used within two weeks of surgical implantation, autogenous fistulae require venous dilatation over a 4-6 week period to allow successful needling for dialysis. Failure of development rather than early thrombosis is a common cause of failure in radiocephalic fistulae. Wong *et al* [3] have shown that measurement of the velocity of flow in the fistula vein at 24 hours, vein size and blood flow at three weeks post-surgery are good predictors of success (Figures 1-4). If the vein remains small and fistula flow low, then duplex scanning, magnetic resonance angiography, brachial arteriography or fistulography may reveal the cause. Such fistulae often have a stenosis in the fistula vein within 2cm of the anastomosis, or arterial stenosis, both of which may be amenable to angioplasty or revisional surgery [6]. If neither option appears feasible then a new AV fistula should be fashioned at a more proximal site. However, it

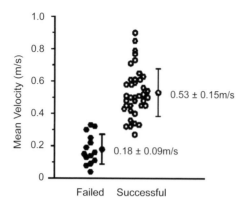

Figure 1 Comparison of AV fistula flow measure by duplex Doppler 24 hours after surgery in failed and successful radiocephalic AV fistulae.

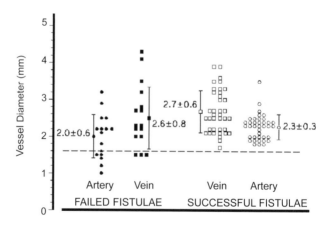

Figure 2 Comparison of arterial and venous diameters in failed and successful AV fistulae.

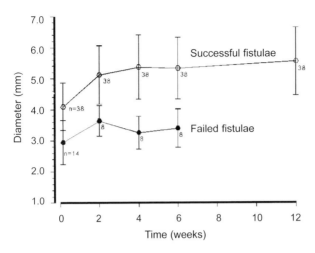

Figure 3 Change in the diameter of the vein draining an AV fistula with time after surgery in failed and successful AV fistulae.

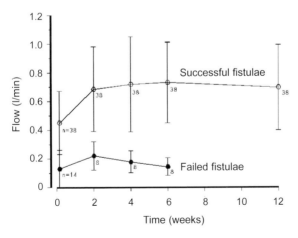

Figure 4 The change in blood flow with time after surgery through failed and successful AV fistulae.

is essential to make an early decision to intervene, preferably within one month, rather than procrastinate, as continued haemodialysis through a central venous catheter increases morbidity.

Late complications

Infection

Infection is a major risk in patients with renal failure and is the second commonest cause of death in uraemic patients after cardiovascular disease. It is most common when there is open access to the circulation as occurs with central venous dialysis catheters. The Dialysis Outcomes and Practice Patterns Study (DOPPS) has shown that temporary catheters have almost an eight times risk of infection and tunnelled catheters, five times the risk of infection compared with fistulae [7], and the risk of sepsis is one of the most potent arguments against their prolonged use for vascular access. The incidence of infectious complications in autogenous AV fistulae remains low at 2-3%. Prosthetic grafts have a nine times higher instance of infection and give rise to the majority of access-related infections requiring surgical intervention. The incidence of infection increases with time and may be as high as 35% during the lifetime of a graft [8].

The commonest organism causing graft infection remains *Staphylococcus aureus*. However, others, such as streptococci and gram-negative bacilli, are significant contributors. Antibiotics should be prescribed on the basis of bacteriological culture and antibiotic sensitivities, although frequently they need to be started on an empirical 'best guess' basis when there is obvious inflammation around a needle puncture site before any discharge occurs. In such cases, flucloxacillin is the first-line treatment, followed by vancomycin. Methicillin-resistant *Staphylococcus aureus* (MRSA) is an increasing problem for which teicoplanin or linezolid is appropriate.

Autogenous fistula infections are infrequent. They often arise as an infected haematoma, which may develop into an abscess requiring formal surgical drainage. Despite cellulitis or abscess formation, autogenous fistulae rarely require ligation. In contrast, graft fistula infections generally do not resolve with antibiotics and usually require either partial or total graft excision. If the infection does not involve either the arterial or venous anastomosis and is confined to one limb of the graft, local excision of the infected segment, with segmental bypass using a new PTFE graft segment may succeed after a period of antibiotic therapy (Figure 5). The author has several patients whose PTFE grafts have been maintained by repeated segmental graft replacement over many years. However, where the infection involves a large segment, the safest policy is to excise the whole graft. In such cases, the vein may be simply ligated, whereas at the arterial end, a very small segment of the graft may be left in place and oversewn in order to avoid narrowing the artery. Alternatively, the whole graft may be taken off the artery and the artery closed with a vein patch.

In those patients with infection close to the arterial anastomosis, the graft must be totally excised. If the arterial anastomosis is actually infected then a vein patch may disrupt, causing major haemorrhage. In this situation the vessel is often very friable and the only solution may be arterial ligation. Whilst this risks acute ischaemia of the hand, limb loss is infrequent, because of the excellent collateral blood supply.

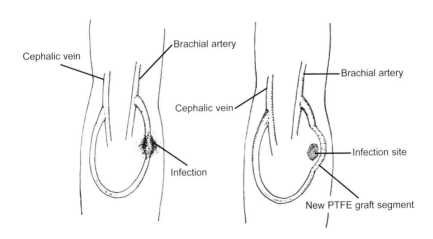

Figure 5 Local excision and bypass of an infected segment of a prosthetic AV loop.

Thrombosis

Despite a significant early failure rate, radiocephalic AV fistulae have an excellent long-term patency of up to 78% at three years [9]. Other more proximal autogenous fistulae have a lower initial failure rate, but a similar long-term outcome. Nevertheless, the commonest complication following AV fistula construction is thrombosis.

Thrombosis is common in patients with prosthetic grafts and is usually associated with either haemodynamic instability or, most frequently, progressive stenosis due to intimal hyperplasia at the venous anastomosis or within the graft at needling sites. The cause of intimal hyperplasia remains unknown, although haemodynamic factors such as wall shear stress have been implicated. Attempts to prevent this by irradiation, photodynamic therapy or drug therapy have been unsuccessful so far, although there is renewed interest in this area. Whilst some grafts remain patent for a long period, most require radiological or surgical intervention at some stage to maintain patency. When no cause for thrombosis can be found, thrombectomy is usually straightforward and oral anticoagulation with warfarin may be warranted. There is little to lose by radiological or surgical intervention for any thrombosed mature fistula and much to gain. Graft thrombectomy can be performed percutaneously, by aspiration, thrombolysis or a mechanical device, e.g. Angiojet, followed by angioplasty. An alternative is surgical thrombectomy with on-table angioplasty performed as a joint procedure.

The Dialysis Outcomes and Quality Initiative (DOQI) [5] guidelines in the US recommend monitoring of graft fistulae to diagnose impending graft failure. A variety of techniques ranging from serial duplex scanning, blood flow measurements and venous pressure measurements during dialysis have been advocated. There is now increasing evidence that surveillance of autogenous AV fistulae using blood flow measurements may be useful (see Chapter 12), but as yet such monitoring has not been generally introduced.

Steal syndrome

Vascular insufficiency of the hand and forearm may occur following proximal AV fistula creation. Reports of hand ischaemia following radiocephalic AV fistula are exceedingly rare, and most cases of peripheral ischaemia relate to brachial fistulae. The first symptoms of steal syndrome may even appear during surgery if local anaesthesia is used. Symptoms of tingling or numbness in the fingers may occur and progress to pain, pallor and coldness of the hand. In severe cases, almost complete loss of sensory and motor nerve function may occur, described as ischaemic monomelic neuropathy. The latter situation is highly dangerous and unless the fistula is reversed or revised within hours, and certainly within 24 hours, then long-term ischaemic damage may result. Fortunately, most cases are less severe and present at later follow-up. A sure sign of steal syndrome is when the patient attends clinic with a single gloved hand on the side of the AV fistula to combat the feeling of coldness!

Steal syndrome occurs in 1.6-8% of brachial AV fistulae [8]. Its incidence is higher in diabetics, who may have disease of the radial and ulnar arteries. Diagnosis can be simply made at the bedside or in the outpatient clinic by using a hand-held continuous wave Doppler probe to measure arterial pressure at the wrist and comparing this with the systemic pressure. Invariably, the wrist brachial pressure index (WBPI), which is analogous to the ankle brachial pressure index (ABPI), is reduced in steal syndrome, invariably to less than 0.6. Another simpler sign of steal syndrome is the presence of a weak or absent radial pulse, which normalises on compressing the fistula. In the worst cases with a very low WBPI, steal may lead to digital gangrene and ulceration (Figure 6), unless

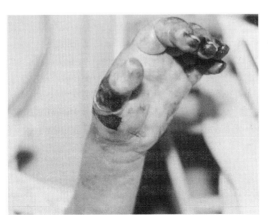

Figure 6 Digital gangrene due to severe steal in a patient with a brachiocephalic AV fistula.

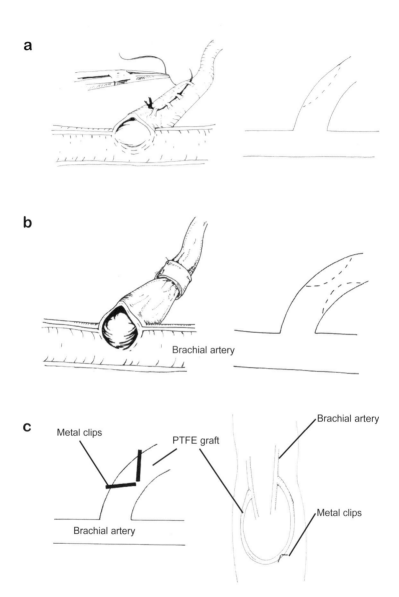

Figure 7 Three techniques to reduce AV fistula flow in steal syndrome by narrowing the outflow: a) using sutures; b) by banding; c) using metallic clips.

surgery is performed to modify or ligate the fistula. In less severe cases, the blood flow may readjust over time so that the WBPI returns to normal.

Apart from the drastic step of ligating the AV fistula, there are several ways to modify the fistula to reduce proximal blood flow and improve distal perfusion. The commonest methods used narrow the lumen of the fistula by sutures, application of metallic clips, banding or the interposition of a narrow segment of PTFE (Figure 7). However, the degree of narrowing is unpredictable and is often either inadequate, with no improvement in symptoms, or excessive, leading to fistula thrombosis. In order to achieve greater success some way of assessing intra-operative digital perfusion must be undertaken. Current techniques include on-table WBPI measurement, needle pressure measurements, digital photoplethys-mography, pulse oximetry, duplex ultrasound and pulse volume recording. However, postoperative symptoms may not always be in keeping with intra-operative findings and hence require close follow-up.

Schanzer *et al* [10] were the first to describe the DRIL (distal ligation with interval ligation) procedure to treat steal syndrome (Figure 8). In this

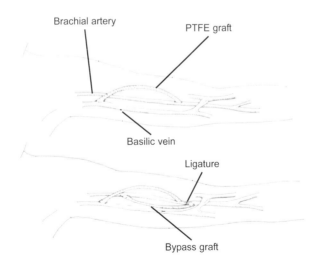

Figure 8 The DRIL procedure for steal syndrome following a PTFE brachiobasilic AV graft showing the positions of the ligature on the brachial artery and the distal bypass.

technique, the brachial artery just distal to the AV fistula is ligated to prevent backflow from the distal artery and a bypass graft is taken from the proximal brachial artery to the artery beyond the ligature to revascularise the hand. The bypass immediately improves blood flow to the hand with resolution of symptoms, but long-term results beyond two years have yet to be published.

Another effective method that the author has used occasionally is to take down the AV fistula, oversew the brachial artery anastomosis and extend the fistula onto the proximal ulnar or radial artery, just distal to the brachial artery bifurcation (the extension procedure) (Figure 9) [11].

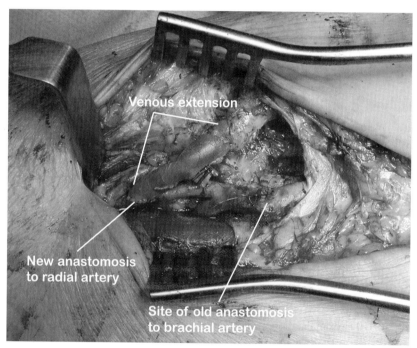

Figure 9 The extension procedure.

This is an easy and satisfactory operation for an autogenous brachiocephalic or brachiobasilic fistula, since the forearm basilic or other adjacent vein can be used. However, the procedure is more difficult for a prosthetic graft.

Another possible procedure for steal in a brachial AV fistula is to detach the vein or graft from the brachial artery and insert a prosthetic graft to it from the axillary artery (proximalisation of the arterial inflow - Figure 10) [12].

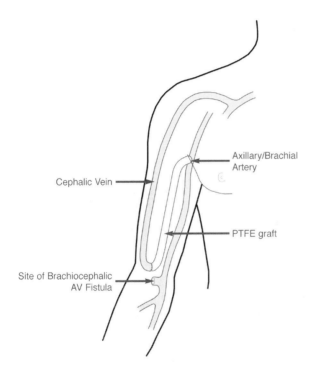

Cephalic Vein

Axillary/Brachial Artery

PTFE graft

Site of Brachiocephalic AV Fistula

Figure 10 Proximalisation of arterial inflow to treat steal syndrome.

Venous hypertension

Venous hypertension can be due to local factors or central venous stenosis. In any radiocephalic AV fistula, particularly those with a side-to-side anastomosis, retrograde venous flow may occur if the valves in either the cephalic vein itself or the dorsal branch of the cephalic vein become incompetent. The flow towards the hand may cause swelling of one or more digits and, even extend to ulceration if longstanding. This problem is more likely to occur if there is a stenosis more proximally in the fistula vein. The problems are usually easily resolved by converting a side-to-side anastomosis to an end-to-side by ligating the distal vein, or ligating the dorsal branch of the cephalic vein and dealing with any stenosis in the main vein by angioplasty.

Following fistula creation, the commonest cause of limb swelling, which usually involves the whole upper limb, is central venous stenosis or occlusion. There is usually a history of subclavian catheterisation but internal jugular catheters can also sometimes cause brachiocephalic vein stenosis. The diagnosis can be confirmed by venography. Treatment options range from percutaneous transluminal angioplasty of the stenosis, with or without stent insertion, or ligation of the fistula. Another option is an internal jugular vein bypass to the subclavian vein distal to the stenosis/occlusion. The internal jugular vein is ligated high in the neck, and mobilised, so that it can be reflected down onto the distal subclavian vein allowing blood to flow from the subclavian vein via the distal internal jugular vein and the brachiocephalic vein into the superior vena cava. Clearly, if there is stenosis in the brachiocephalic vein then this technique is not feasible.

The high risk of subclavian stenosis is the main reason to avoid subclavian vein catheterisation, as this may preclude an ipsilateral AV fistula.

Cardiac failure due to high blood flow in AV fistulae

The flow through an AV fistula normally ranges from 500-1000ml/min, but this may reach several litres/minute in more proximal fistulae. With very high flows, heart failure may occur. The diagnosis may be confirmed by a reduction in heart rate following temporary occlusion of the fistula (Branham's sign). The treatment is either fistula ligation with the creation of another in the opposite arm or to attempt to reduce its flow rate.

Surgical banding with either sutures or interposition of a short segment of PTFE graft has variable success because of the difficulty in quantifying the effect intra-operatively. An alternative option is to transfer the arterial inflow to a more distal site, e.g. radial or ulnar artery, using a bridging graft.

Neuropathy

The most severe acute neurological complication after fistula surgery is monomelic ischaemic neuropathy. This is associated with steal syndrome and is characterised by severe sensorimotor nerve dysfunction, typically occurring within hours of fistula creation. Unless the fistula is reversed immediately, the neuronal ischaemia may result in permanent damage, which cannot be reversed by later revascularisation.

Carpal tunnel syndrome is thought to occur more frequently in limbs with AV fistula patients. The cause of these symptoms, however, remains uncertain, but may be due to median nerve compression by oedema within the carpal tunnel. Nerve conduction studies should confirm a decrease in nerve conduction velocity. A release of the flexor retinaculum will resolve the symptoms.

Aneurysms

A false aneurysm usually results from perforation of the back wall of the fistula by the dialysis needle with persistent bleeding to produce an expansile haematoma. A duplex scan will reveal an arterial jet into the haematoma. Surgical evacuation of the haematoma and oversewing of the bleeding site is usually all that is required. Aneurysm formation in a mature fistula may be due to proximal venous stenosis, which can be detected by a duplex scan. Angioplasty may arrest further dilatation and allow needling of a proximal fistula segment.

True aneurysmal dilatation of the vein draining an AV fistula is not uncommon in longstanding dialysis patients. Provided there is no risk of ulceration at the needle puncture site, intervention is not required. However, the fistula can be cosmetically unacceptable, especially to young women. In such cases, creating a fistula in the other arm and, when mature, excising the aneurysmal fistula is most appropriate.

Seroma

A seroma is a sterile collection of crystalline fluid with a high protein content contained in a non-secretory fibrous pseudomembrane, which may be localised around a graft. Its aetiology remains unknown. If limited in extent, the avoidance of the affected segment for dialysis may be all that is required. However, if the seroma is more extensive, drainage is worth trying but graft excision may be required for complete resolution.

Conclusions

Vascular access is potentially associated with many complications immediately after surgical creation and much later. The very need for the fistula to be needled for dialysis in the long term, makes access surgery unique amongst vascular surgical procedures. A case can be made for surgeons to monitor patients in the outpatient clinic in order to pick up problems early, as with other vascular operations, rather than waiting for renal units to report them. Vascular access surgery is vital to the life and well-being of dialysis patients. Patients in established renal failure are already considerably disadvantaged by the need for dialysis and the least that can be expected by them is for access complications to be monitored and dealt with expeditiously by the multidisciplinary team.

Acknowledgements

Thanks are due to Mr Geoffrey Owen, former Research Nurse in the Transplant Unit, for figures 5, 7 and 8. Figures 1-4 are derived from the paper by Wong *et al* [3], with permission from the journal *European Journal of Vascular and Endovascular Surgery*. Thanks are also due to Gill Rycroft in the Medical Illustration Department of the Royal Liverpool University Hospital for Figure 10.

Key Summary

◆ Autogenous AV fistulae have the best long-term patency.

◆ Thrombosis of AV fistulae is the commonest long-term complication, particularly if prosthetic grafts are used. There is evidence that screening of graft fistulae may predict thrombosis.

◆ Infection risk is higher in graft fistulae than autogenous AV fistulae.

◆ Steal syndrome can occur in fistulae with arterial inflow from the brachial artery. Any patient with pain and coldness in the hand following such a fistula is likely to have steal and needs to be investigated, monitored carefully and appropriate surgery performed.

◆ Cardiac failure may occur in patients with high-flow fistulae.

References

1. Cheesbrough, JS, Finch RG, Burden RP. A prospective study of the mechanisms of infection associated with haemodialysis catheters. *J Infect Dis* 1986; 154: 579-89.

2. Pruett TL. *Vascular access infections in vascular access for haemodialysis* VII. Henry ML, Ed. Precept Press, 2001.

3. Wong V, Ward R, Taylor J, *et al.* Factors associated with early failure of arteriovenous fistulae for haemodialysis access. *Eur J Vasc Endovasc Surg* 1996; 12: 207-13.

4. Lemson MS, Leunissen KM, Tordoir JH. Does pre-operative duplex examination improve patency rates of Brescia-Cimino fistulas? *Nephrol Dial Transplant* 1998; 13: 1360-1.

5. NKF-DOQI. Clinical practice guidelines for vascular access. *Am J Kidney Disease* 1997; 30: 5150-91.

6.   Turmel-Rodrigues L, Pengloan J, Bauidin S, *et al*. Treatment of stenosis and thrombosis in haemodialysis fistula and grafts by interventional radiology. *Nephrol Dial Transplant* 2000; 15: 2029-36.

7.   Rayner HC, Pisoni RL, Gillespie BW, *et al*. Creation, cannulation and survival of arteriovenous fistulae - Data from the Dialysis Outcomes and Practice Patterns Study. *Kidney Int* 2003; 63: 323-30.

8.   Zibari GB, Rohr MS, Landreneau MD, *et al*. Complications from permanent haemodialysis vascular access. *Surgery* 1998; 104: 681-6.

9.   Mehta S. Statistical summary of clinical results of vascular access procedures for haemodialysis. In: *Vascular Access for Haemodialysis*, 2nd Edition. Sommer BG, Henry ML, Eds. Precept Press, Inc., 1991: 145-57.

10.   Schanzer H, Schwartz M, Harrington E, *et al*. Treatment of ischemia due to 'steal' by arteriovenous fistula with distal artery ligation and revascularization. *J Vasc Surg* 1988; 7: 770-3.

11.   Ehsan O, Bhattacharya D, Darwish A, *et al*. 'Extension technique': a modified technique for brachio-cephalic fistula to prevent dialysis access-associated steal syndrome. *Eur J Vasc Endovasc Surg* 2005; 29: 324-7.

12.   Zanow J, Kruger U, Scholtz H. Proximalization of the arterial inflow - a new technique to treat access-related ischaemia. *J Vasc Surg* 2006; 43: 1216-21.

Chapter 11

Infection and vascular access

Peter Choi MA MB PhD MRCP, *Consultant Nephrologist*
Andrew H Frankel BSc MB BS MD FRCP, *Consultant Nephrologist*
West London Renal and Transplant Centre, Hammersmith Hospital, London, UK

Introduction

The major complication of vascular access and particularly haemodialysis catheters relates to their associated incidence of infection, which can be described as the Achilles heel of dialysis treatment. This increased risk of infection is contributed to by multiple factors, including acquired defects in neutrophil function of dialysis patients, the presence of non-biological material used for dialysis access, the breaks in the skin associated with this access and the many manoeuvres required for the dialysis procedure itself. The surveillance study by the US Centre for Disease Control [1], monitoring more than 150,000 patient-months of haemodialysis treatment, confirmed the high rate of infection associated with dialysis vascular access and particularly with haemodialysis catheters, as compared to arteriovenous (AV) fistulae and grafts (Table 1).

The incidence of infection is greater for non-tunnelled, as opposed to tunnelled catheters and is related to the duration of placement. With regard to tunnelled catheters, Tesio catheters have been reported to have low associated infection rates, and this has led some units to use them routinely for long-term haemodialysis access [2].

Infection can present in a number of ways, including localised infection at the catheter exit site, over the graft or AV fistula, or as a systemic bacteraemia with metastatic infection. Systemic bacteraemia is characterised by fever, leucocytosis and an inflammatory response, and distant spread from a catheter or graft infection is not uncommon and is

Table 1 Event rate for infectious complications by access type. Dialysis Surveillance Network, October 1999-May 2001 [1].

	Autogenous fistulae	Prosthetic graft	Tunnelled catheter	Non-tunnelled catheter	All access
Access infections (events)	130	421	1594	284	2429
Access infections (event rate per 100 patient-months)	0.56	1.36	8.42	11.98	3.2

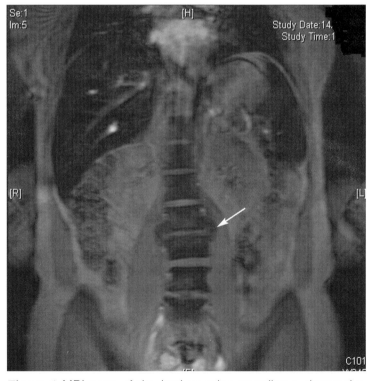

Figure 1 MRI scan of the lumbar spine revealing a destructive osteomyelitis (arrow) in a patient with a history of a *Staphylococcus aureus* bacteraemia from a tunnelled catheter.

associated with significant morbidity and mortality (Figure 1). Types of metastatic infection include:

- septic thrombosis of central veins;
- septic pulmonary emboli;
- acute endocarditis;
- osteomyelitis;
- septic arthritis;
- shock and death.

The incidence of these infective complications of vascular access is not insignificant and in an audit across London renal units there were a substantial number of these complications. As one would predict, the incidence of these complications varied with the percentage of patients who are dialysed by non-tunnelled haemodialysis catheters (Table 2).

Table 2 Incidence of specific infective complications of vascular access, related to the percentage of long-term haemodialysis patients using temporary non-tunnelled dialysis catheters. Data were collected over two months (September-October 2002) in renal units across London (anonymously denoted A-G).

Unit	% Temporary catheters	Number of cases				
		Systemic sepsis	Infective endocarditis	Osteomyelitis	Other	Death
A	0	8	0	0	0	0
C	0	1	0	0	0	0
B	1	21	1	1	1	3
E	1	24	0	0	1	1
G	3	11	1	1	1	2
F	9	68	2	2	3	2
D	11	6	0	0	0	1

Non-tunnelled haemodialysis catheters have the highest risk of infection and the intensive care unit (ICU) experience can be used to identify the factors which determine the risks for such an infection. Within the ICU literature the risk of infection relates to the site of insertion of the non-tunnelled line, with the greatest risk occurring with femoral vein catheters, followed by internal jugular and then subclavian catheters. Furthermore, the site of insertion influences the natural history and presentation of infection, with the majority of infections occurring within one week of insertion of femoral catheters, while internal jugular and subclavian catheter infections peak around three weeks following insertion. In a study by Oliver *et al* [3], 5.4% of temporary non-tunnelled internal jugular catheters became infected after three weeks and 10.7% of femoral catheters became infected after one week. The subclavian route is contraindicated as a route for placement of haemodialysis catheters because of the high associated incidence of central vein stenosis. Furthermore, specific groups of patients are recognised to be at increased risk of catheter infection (Table 3).

Table 3 Patient factors associated with an increased risk of haemodialysis catheter infection.

- Chronic carriage of bacteria

- Patients with stomas (tracheostomy, urotomy, colostomy)

- Diabetics

- Hypo-albuminaemic patients

- Non-compliant patients

- Elderly

Infection associated with vascular access has considerable cost, both to the patient and the health economy. Catheters may need to be removed and there is an incidence of infection-associated thrombosis of major veins. Patients often require hospitalisation and access-related infection is one of the commonest causes of admission for haemodialysis patients. In the 2002 survey of London renal units, incident haemodialysis patients were monitored over a two-month period for infectious complications and admissions. There were no hospital admissions due to infective complications in new patients using AV fistulae as their primary access. In contrast, 894 patient-days were lost to infective complications from tunnelled and non-tunnelled haemodialysis catheters. The number of patient-days per unit correlated most significantly with the percentage of their total dialysis population using non-tunnelled haemodialysis catheters.

Prevention of infection

There is considerable pressure on all renal units to undertake a program aimed at reducing the incidence of infection. The implementation of a multidisciplinary team approach in dialysis catheter care has been shown to improve patient outcomes [4]. From the data already described it is clear that measures aimed to reduce the use of all types of haemodialysis catheters will be important in reducing infection rates and therefore, all aspects of good vascular access practice, including early referral and planning for long-term haemodialysis access, should be implemented.

There are two routes by which infection can occur in patients with haemodialysis catheters:

◆ infection or colonisation at the exit site, followed by spread down the outside of the catheter, resulting in either a tunnel infection in those with tunnelled lines, or blood-borne infection in those with non-tunnelled lines;
◆ spread along the inner wall of the catheter.

Prevention of infection should be directed to each of these two portals of entry and a number of guidelines and recommendations have been produced in this rapidly developing field [5].

Scrupulous aseptic care, at the time of insertion is vital and use of prophylactic antibiotics is of particular relevance to patients who are undergoing insertion of a tunnelled catheter. The colonisation of the exit site is associated with an increased risk of subsequent bacteraemia, usually by a similar organism to that present at the exit site. Therefore, non-specific measures to maintain a clean and infection-free exit site may be associated with a reduction in systemic infection rates. Haemodialysis catheter dressings should be changed at each haemodialysis session, using an aseptic technique. The exit site should be inspected for signs of infection and swabs should be taken if there is any evidence of a discharge. The area should be cleaned with an appropriate antiseptic and there is evidence suggesting that the use of chlorhexidine or povidone-iodine reduces the risk of exit-site infections and subsequent septicaemia. Levin *et al* [6] demonstrated that cleaning exit sites with povidone-iodine, rather than normal saline, reduced exit-site infection rates from 18% to 5% and systemic sepsis rates from 17% to 2%. The use of alcohol-containing cleaning fluids on some dialysis catheters may damage the catheter. However, this is less important for patients who require temporary haemodialysis catheters for short periods of time and is of more pertinence to long-term tunnelled haemodialysis catheters. Therefore, all non-tunnelled catheters, which are likely to be in place for less than a week, should be cleaned with povidine-iodine or alcohol-based solution and tunnelled catheters in use should only be those that are able to be cleaned by similar agents.

Mucocutaneous colonisation with specific gram-positive bacteria, such as *Staphylococcus aureus* (*S. aureus*), is associated with an increased risk of exit-site infection and subsequent blood-borne infection. *S. aureus* is the most significant organism associated with central venous catheter infections and is highly virulent, frequently leading to osteomyelitis and endocarditis, which can be aggressive and difficult to treat. (The question of methicillin sensitivity is of relevance only to the treatment, but not to the morbidity.) Because of this, colonisation should be routinely assessed and treated. Intranasal mupirocin cream should be used for nasal carriers of *S. aureus*, and has been shown to be of benefit to patients with tunnelled PD catheters [7].

The application of mupirocin to the exit site to prevent exit-site colonisation with *S. aureus* and staphylococcal septicaemia has been controversial, but there are now studies to recommend its routine use. In a study of patients with tunnelled catheters, Johnson *et al* [8] showed that compared with controls, mupirocin-treated patients experienced significantly fewer catheter-related bacteraemias (7 vs 35%, p<0.01) and a longer time to first bacteraemia. The beneficial effect of mupirocin was entirely attributable to a reduction in staphylococcal infection (log rank 10.69, p=0.001) and was still observed when only patients without prior nasal *S. aureus* carriage were included in the analysis. There has been concern that this practice could result in mupirocin resistance, but this seems to have a low incidence in practice and remains clinically unimportant. Moreover, there does not appear to be any increase in non-staphylococcal infections.

Colonisation of the internal wall of the catheter is a frequent occurrence and is usually associated with the presence of a biofilm. This is produced by a combination of host factors (e.g. fibrinogen and fibrin) and microbial products (e.g. glycocalyx). Within the biofilm the colonising bacteria convert to a sessile form and live in symbiosis with the patient. Colonisation of the luminal wall occurs within 12-24 hours of insertion of most catheters. The colonising organism is frequently not identified by standard microbiological tests and the reasons for the subsequent development of overt infection in a particular individual are poorly defined. There appears to be a link between the number of organisms retrieved by culture from the catheter surface and the risk of infection.

Impregnation of the catheters with antibacterial agents, such as silver or antibiotics has been used to try and reduce the incidence of catheter-associated infections. This manoeuvre has been found to reduce the incidence of infections, particularly in ITU, but carries risks of patient sensitivity and the development of bacterial resistance. Antibiotic impregnation has been utilised mainly for non-tunnelled catheters and has been associated with a significant reduction in infection in the short term [9].

Locking the catheters with antibiotic solutions has also been tried, and there is evidence to support gentamicin, cefotaxime and minocycline antibiotic lock strategies. This technique is of benefit in reducing the rate of infection with both tunnelled and non-tunnelled catheters [10]. Concerns of resistance and toxicity have so far proven to be unfounded.

Aside from antibiotic locks, antibacterial agents that have antithrombotic action have been utilised as an alternative to standard heparin locks. Citrate in high concentrations on its own or accompanied by Taurolidine has been tried and there is some evidence supporting its use and a reduction in the incidence of septicaemia or bacteraemia, but not exit-site colonisation and infection [11]. This approach is supported by evidence that the catheter lock solution can influence the biology of the biofilm and that while heparin may enhance formation of some biofilms, sodium citrate or EDTA as a catheter lock may inhibit biofilm formation [12]. Further studies are required before either of these techniques can be recommended for routine use with tunnelled catheters.

In order for an individual unit to be able to make judgements about their own policies, it is vital that they have knowledge throughout their organisation of their infection rates for different forms of vascular access. Adequate information on infection rates within individual units provides an important stimulus to introducing changes in practice, aimed at reducing the rate of infection. Therefore, proper surveillance and audit, documenting infection episodes per standard unit of catheter time (most usually per thousand days of catheter usage) should be undertaken at each unit.

Treatment of infection

Treatment of access-related infection depends on access type and the site of infection. In general, the treatment of non-tunnelled catheter infection is based upon a low threshold for catheter removal, given the temporary nature of such access. Significant exit-site infection in a non-tunnelled catheter should prompt consideration for its removal. Where there is evidence of blood-borne infection in patients with temporary lines, the catheter should be removed at the earliest opportunity.

In contrast, the treatment of infection associated with a tunnelled catheter or graft involves a greater consideration of a patient's previous access history and the availability of subsequent access routes. For tunnelled catheters and infected grafts, the diagnosis must be accurately made by appropriate cultures (including cultures taken from the lines) and appropriate imaging. Tunnelled catheters are more difficult to change, particularly in patients in whom sites for access are limited. In these situations, initial empiric antibiotic regimes should be started and the catheter only removed if markers of infection (fever, white cell count and CRP) fail to improve on this regime. Catheters and grafts may be salvageable, although a prolonged antibiotic course is often required (six weeks). The presence of persistently positive blood cultures, despite appropriate antibiotics, should prompt immediate removal of the line and a search for potential sites of metastatic infection.

Antibiotic use should be judicious and take into account both national guidelines and local resistance patterns, to reduce the development of antibiotic resistance. In general, exit-site infection may be treated with topical agents and/or oral antibiotics, but severe infection and catheter-associated bacteraemia, require empiric intravenous broad-spectrum antibiotics. Gram-positive organisms account for the majority of access-related infections; however, the range of organisms will vary and may be influenced by the interventions adopted locally to prevent access-related infection. A broad-based regime should include vancomycin and an appropriate intravenous gram-negative agent. If there is evidence of associated soft tissue infection around the tunnel or around the graft, penetrative antibiotics (rifampicin or fucidin if gram-positive organisms suspected) should be included in the chosen regime.

Conclusions

Infection associated with vascular access remains a major challenge to all those involved in the care of patients with end-stage renal failure. The management of this problem requires a program aimed at reducing the incidence to the absolute minimum and treating those who develop infection in a planned manner. Many simple manouevres can be utilised to reduce the infection risk; however, the most important intervention is a strategic commitment to reduction in infection across all staff who work within an individual unit.

Key Summary

◆ Infection is the main complication of vascular access and carries with it significant patient morbidity and mortality.

◆ While the native arteriovenous fistulae carry the lowest incidence of infection of any form of access, catheters and grafts are still likely to be required and the incidence of infection when using these forms of access can be reduced.

◆ In order to reduce the incidence of infection units must first have a clear knowledge of their infection rates.

◆ Haemodialysis exit sites should be regularly cleaned with antiseptic agents and have aseptic dressing changes at each dialysis. Mupirocin on the exit site should be considered in units that have a high incidence of *Staphylococcus aureus* infections.

◆ Antibiotic-coated lines can reduce the rate of infection associated with non-tunnelled lines and antibacterial locks can reduce the infection rates for tunnelled haemodialysis catheters.

◆ Infection in a non-tunnelled catheter should prompt consideration of removal of the catheter and appropriate antibiotic therapy.

◆ Tunnelled lines and grafts may be the only form of access for some patients and therefore strategies should be aimed at preservation of these forms of access. This should include clear guidleines for the treatment of access-associated infection.

References

1. Tokars JI, Miller ER, Stein G. New national surveillance system for haemodialysis-associated infections: initial results. *AJIC* 2002; 30: 288-95.

2. Duncan ND, Singh S, Cairns TD, *et al*. Tesio-Caths provide effective and safe long-term vascular access. *Nephrol Dial Transplant* 2004; 19: 2816-22.

3. Oliver MJ, Callery SM, Thorpe KE, *et al*. Risk of bacteraemia from temporary haemodialysis catheters by site of insertion and duration of use: a prospective study. *Kidney Int* 2000; 58: 2543-5.

4. Mokrzycki MH, Zhang M, Golestaneh L, *et al*. An interventional controlled trial comparing 2 management models for the treatment of tunnelled catheter bacteraemia: a collaborative team model versus usual physician managed care. *Am J Kidney Dis* 2006; 48: 587-95.

5. Guidelines for preventing infections associated with the insertion and maintenance of central venous catheters. *Journal of Hospital Infection* 2001; 47(Supplement): S47-S 67.

6. Levin A, Mason AJ, Jindal KK, *et al*. Prevention of haemodialysis subclavian vein catheter infections by topical povidone-iodine. *Kidney Int* 1991; 40: 934-8.

7. Mupirocin Study Group. Nasal mupirocin prevents *Staphylococcus aureus* exit-site infection during peritoneal dialysis. *J Am Soc Nephrol* 1996; 7: 2403-8.

8. Johnson DW, Macginley R, Kay TD, *et al*. A randomized controlled trial of topical exit-site mupirocin application in patients with tunnelled, cuffed haemodialysis catheters. *Nephrol Dial Transplant* 2002; 17: 1802-7.

9. Bambauer R, Mestres P, Schiel R, *et al*. Surface-treated large bore catheters with silver-based coatings versus untreated catheters for extracorporeal detoxification methods. *ASAIO J* 1998; 44: 303-8.

10. McIntyre CW, Hulme LJ, Taal M, Fluck RJ. Locking of tunnelled haemodialysis catheters with gentamicin and heparin. *Kidney Int* 2004; 66: 801-5.

11. Betjes MG, Van Agteren M. Prevention of dialysis access-related sepsis with citrate-Taurolidine containing lock solution. *Nephrol Dial Transplant* 2004; 19: 1546-51.

12. Shanks RM, Sargent JL, Martinez RM, *et al*. Catheter lock solutions influence staphylococcal biofilm formation on abiotic surfaces. *Nephrol Dial Transplant* 2006; 21: 2247-55.

Chapter 12
Function and surveillance

Alison J Armitage MB ChB MRCP MD, *Senior Registrar in Nephrology*

Charles RV Tomson MA BM BCh FRCP DM (Oxon), *Consultant Nephrologist*

Southmead Hospital, Bristol, UK

Introduction

Sudden failure of an arteriovenous (AV) fistula or a PTFE graft can represent a disaster for a dialysis patient, involving hospitalisation, attempts (usually unsuccessful) to restore flow using massage, thrombolytics, or thrombectomy, placement of temporary venous catheters with their associated risks, and construction of a new fistula or graft at another site. The suggestion that thrombosis can be predicted by routine surveillance to detect stenoses, and prevented by timely intervention with angioplasty or surgical revision, is therefore appealing. In this chapter we review the evidence that routine surveillance, using non-invasive methods to predict incipient thrombosis and allow pre-emptive correction of the underlying problem, helps to reduce access failure. Because the risk of thrombosis is so much higher in grafts than in fistulae, most of the available evidence relates to grafts. There are major differences in the cause of failure of the two types of access, and so evidence cannot safely be extrapolated to fistulae. Studies that have combined both types of access need to be interpreted with caution.

Causes of access failure

The great majority of PTFE grafts fail due to thrombosis at a stenosis either along the graft or near the venous anastomosis. These stenoses are caused by intimal hyperplasia. A small number fail secondary to infection or require ligation for acute haemorrhage. Early failure of AV fistulae, in contrast, is most commonly because of poor flow due to poor inflow or stenosis at or just beyond the anastomosis. AV fistulae, once established, are much less likely to fail than PTFE grafts; when failure occurs it may be due to complications of aneurysmal dilatation of the fistula or to infection, as well as intimal hyperplasia. Virchow's triad of risk factors for thrombosis comprises abnormalities in blood flow, abnormal blood constituents, and abnormal vessel wall. In the case of thrombosed fistulae or grafts, abnormalities in blood flow appear to be the most important risk factor. Every time a fistula or graft is needled there is endothelial damage, and cessation of bleeding after withdrawal of the needles requires thrombosis to occur at that site, but if there is high flow through the access thrombus is prevented from propagating into the lumen. Thrombosis is much more common within grafts than within established fistulae, but it is unclear how much this is due to recognition of the wall of PTFE grafts as foreign and how much to the increased prevalence of stenoses causing reduced and turbulent flow. Risk factors for vascular disease such as inherited thrombophilias, anticardiolipin antibodies, dyslipidaemias, chronic inflammation, hyperhomocystinaemia, and acquired anti-thrombin antibodies may contribute to access failure [1], but the great majority of episodes of access thrombosis occur in the absence of any such abnormalities. There is no good evidence that systemic anticoagulation reduces the risk. The evidence that antiplatelet agents reduce the risk of access thrombosis is limited, and confounded by the observation that dipyridamole, but not other antiplatelet agents [2], may inhibit vascular smooth muscle proliferation in addition to its effects on platelets. Smoking is a proven risk factor for failure of AV fistulae [3].

Determinants of blood flow through fistulae and grafts

The measurement of venous pressure or of blood flow through a fistula or graft requires understanding of the possible confounding factors influencing these measurements. Simple fluid dynamics predict that the flow (Q_a) through a PTFE graft can be predicted by the pressure drop across the graft and by the resistance (R) across the vascular circuit that carries the blood flow [4]:

$$Q_a = (MAP - CVP)/R$$

(MAP = mean arterial pressure; CVP = central venous pressure)

Grafts and fistulae bypass the arterioles that govern peripheral vascular resistance, and blood flow through them is therefore much less dependent on the degree of peripheral vasoconstriction or vasodilatation than blood flow through other organs. It is therefore illogical to blame access thrombosis on hypovolaemia, if the systemic blood pressure remains normal or high. Indeed, a low CVP with no change in MAP will actually increase the pressure drop across the access and increase flow. Excessive removal of fluid on dialysis can, however, result in a rise in haematocrit and thus of whole blood viscosity, which is one of the determinants of R, although dialysis does not cause sufficient change in haematocrit to have a detectable effect on access blood flow under normal conditions [5].

Low systemic blood pressure is an important cause of low blood flow through access. Extracellular volume is an important determinant of systemic blood pressure in dialysis patients, and an inappropriately low target weight is therefore a potential contributor. Perhaps the most common scenario is an obese patient who continues to gain weight on dialysis, but whose target weight is not revised upwards. The other important cause of hypotension amongst dialysis patients is cardiac failure. Because excess extracellular fluid can be removed on dialysis, this often occurs without the physical signs of oedema and raised venous pressure seen in non-dialysis patients. Low flow may also be caused by reduced pressure in the arterial limb of a fistula or graft, resulting from an inflow stenosis. This can be detected by comparison of the arterial pressure in the graft (during temporary manual occlusion downstream of the needle) with the mean arterial blood pressure in the contralateral arm; a pressure difference of >20mm Hg is highly predictive of an arterial stenosis [6].

Early recognition of the access at risk

Clinical suspicion

Simple palpation and auscultation over a fistula or graft is sometimes sufficient to allow recognition of impending thrombosis. However, fistulae (and, to a lesser extent, grafts) vary enormously from patient to patient and neither the extent of venous distension (visible or palpable), nor the loudness of the vascular bruit heard correlate at all well with blood flow or the risk of subsequent thrombosis. Simple clinical inspection certainly allows monitoring of the development of a newly placed fistula. Sometimes a stenosis can be suspected clinically because of a sudden transition from venous engorgement and a strong thrill to a minimally distended vein with little or no palpable thrill. A change in the degree of distension of a fistula reported by the patient or dialysis nurse should be taken seriously.

Severe upstream stenosis, for instance caused by subclavian vein stenosis, often causes marked venous distension and oedema in the arm below the narrowing. The presence of enlarged collateral veins over the chest wall in such a patient indicates longstanding subclavian stenosis or occlusion and should be further investigated.

Difficulty in placing needles clearly depends on the skill of the person attempting this - usually the patient or a dialysis nurse. To a large extent this is a pragmatic issue: if the most skilled staff member available cannot reliably place two adequately sized needles for dialysis, then the fistula or graft is unsuitable for dialysis, and requires revision, which in turn requires identification of the cause of the problem. Nurses often report aspiration of soft, fresh blood clots from the fistula or graft following attempted needle placement. Thrombus organises rapidly and becomes adherent to the vessel wall, so in this situation clots must be forming on the end of the needle soon after insertion. This may be due to placement of the needle tip at a steep angle to the direction of blood flow, or to some other cause of turbulent flow within the access. Prolonged bleeding after removal of dialysis needles is also frequently seen in patients with an outflow stenosis. However, there are other causes, including, for instance, needling through sites where the skin is thin and atrophic, through false aneurysms in fistulae or through defects in the wall of a PTFE graft. Recently constructed fistulae or grafts are more likely to thrombose than long-established ones [7], as are fistulae or grafts placed in a patient with a previous history of access failure and those which have already required surgical or angiographic intervention.

Decreased adequacy of dialysis

The efficiency with which a dialysis session removes low-molecular-weight uraemic toxins is an important determinant of outcome and is routinely measured - usually on a monthly basis - by calculation either of the Urea Reduction Ratio (URR) or Kt/Vurea. URR is the fractional reduction of

[urea] which occurs during a dialysis treatment, and is a simpler measurement. Kt/V is the dimensionless ratio between the volume cleared of urea and the total distribution volume of urea, and incorporates loss of urea by convection as well as by diffusive exchange. The relative merits of the various methods for calculation of these indices, and the influence of the precise method by which the post-dialysis blood sample is obtained have been reviewed elsewhere [8]. Both are influenced by blood flow, dialyser surface area, dialysate flow, and dialysis time. A fall in URR or Kt/V may be due to many reasons including failure to achieve prescribed blood flow as a result of poor access flow, or to recirculation (discussed below) and may be the first indication of impending access failure. Due to the number of factors influencing it, a change in dialysis adequacy alone is not a reliable enough indicator to be used in the surveillance of vascular access.

Measures of recirculation

The term 'recirculation' refers to a reduction in the efficiency of dialysis caused by blood that has just been returned from the dialysis circuit re-entering the circuit rather than returning to the patient's circulation. Severe recirculation can be caused by an upstream fistula stenosis, or by inadvertent misplacement of the dialysis needles, with the 'arterial' needle being placed upstream of the 'venous' needle. Some 'physiological' recirculation also occurs because of differential perfusion of different body compartments during dialysis due, for instance, to reduced muscle and splanchnic blood flow. Most dialysis units do not routinely measure recirculation, and many of the older methods used may give misleading results. A reduction in efficiency of dialysis results in a fall in URR or Kt/V, and often also in severe pre-dialysis hyperkalaemia, and may occasionally be the first evidence of imminent access failure, particularly if this is causing turbulent, non-linear flow and recirculation within the fistula or graft. However, mid-graft stenosis can easily be missed if reliance is placed on measures of recirculation, as it causes neither recirculation nor high pressures in the venous return line.

Assessment of venous (outflow) pressure

Based on clinical observations that patients whose grafts failed due to upstream stenosis had unusually high venous pressures detected during dialysis, several groups have studied the use of routine measurements of venous pressure in the prediction of the presence of venous stenosis or of access failure [9-20]. Measurement of venous pressures in fistulae is less predictive of upstream stenosis because of the development of collateral branches that form in response to stenoses, with a resultant decrease (or absence of an increase) in pressure. Accurate measurement of venous pressure in the access requires attention to detail. Variations in mean arterial pressure (MAP) contribute to changes in intra-access pressure (P_{IA}), and venous pressure measurements are usually therefore expressed as a ratio of P_{IA}/MAP. Resistance in the tubing and venous needle may contribute variably to venous pressure, depending on blood flow. Pressure measurements taken in the drip chamber also require correction for the height difference between the pressure transducer and the drip chamber (which varies from machine to machine) and that between the drip chamber and the armrest of the dialysis chair [12]. These problems may be avoided by use of a pressure transducer inserted into the venous line close to the venous needle, but this requires extra equipment and is not suitable for routine clinical use [10]. 'Static' venous pressure measurements are taken during conditions of zero flow with a clamp between the dialyser and the drip chamber. P_{IA}/MAP ratios of >0.5 have been found to be associated with significantly reduced blood flow compared to lower ratios [12]. 'Dynamic' venous pressure monitoring was first described by Schwab [9] and involves the measurement of pressure in the drip chamber at a blood flow rate of 200-225ml/minute during the first 30 minutes of dialysis. A venous pressure of >150mm Hg, as measured by the dialysis machine without correction for height of the drip chamber above the patient or other such variables, and irrespective of inflow or mean arterial pressure, was considered abnormal and prompted further investigation with a view to angioplasty or surgery. Numerous groups have subsequently reported the use of dynamic pressure monitoring in the selection of patients for further investigation into possible outflow stenoses [11, 13].

Measured access flow

Numerous techniques have been reported for the direct measurement of access flow, including ultrasound dilution, conductance dilution, haematocrit dilution, thermal dilution, Doppler ultrasound, and magnetic resonance imaging. These techniques have been reviewed in detail elsewhere [1]. All involve measurement of dilution of an indicator, which is dependent upon blood flow. The most widely studied technique is ultrasound dilution [14], which requires reversal of the blood lines together with a bolus injection of saline into the venous line. Sensors on both lines measure the velocity of transmission of ultrasound waves through blood, allowing detection of dilution caused by the saline injection. This technique has become commercially available (Transonic® Systems Inc.), and numerous reports of the use of this technique in identification of patients with low access blood flow, or falling flow over time, have now been published [11, 13, 15]. Most studies involved patients with grafts, but recent studies have shown that patients with native AV fistulae may also benefit from surveillance using measurements of access flow [16, 21-24]. Studies have used receiver operating characteristic (ROC) curves to evaluate the predictive accuracy of a blood flow measurement. For a measurement to be clinically useful it needs to have both a high sensitivity and a low false positive rate for predicting thrombosis or access failure. ROC curves test this by comparing these two variables and by calculation of the area under the curve to ascertain the accuracy of blood flow measurements [7].

Duplex ultrasound scanning

This technique has become the gold standard for initial assessment of fistulae and grafts, and permits simultaneous estimation of blood flow and imaging of stenoses, but is much more expensive than either venous pressure monitoring or ultrasound dilution measurement of access blood flow. Estimation of blood flow is done by multiplying velocity of blood flow by cross-sectional area, and is much more accurate in grafts, where there is less variation in cross-sectional area, than in fistulae. Stenoses are detected by a combination of imaging of vein or graft diameter and measurement of the velocity of blood flow above and below the stenosis. Agreement between estimates of blood flow using duplex ultrasound and those using ultrasound dilution has been reported to be good in one study, in which analysis was confined to patients with PTFE grafts [17], but less good in a recent study in which as many patients had fistulae as grafts [18]. Another study showed that Doppler ultrasound correlated closely to fistulography in diagnosing anatomical stenosis and therefore may be useful to confirm stenoses detected by other methods of monitoring prior to referral for invasive fistulography [19]. In particularly high-risk PTFE grafts it may be reasonable to use this more labour-intensive (and costly) technique as the primary method of surveillance, with duplex scans every 2-3 months.

Clearly, other techniques, such as magnetic resonance angiography and direct angiography, allow detection of anatomical stenoses as well as allowing some assessment of blood flow. However, these techniques are unlikely ever to become used for routine surveillance.

The effectiveness of surveillance methods

Several studies have compared venous pressure monitoring with blood flow monitoring. An example is a study performed by Bosman *et al* [20]. This was a cross-sectional study of 71 forearm PTFE grafts in 42 patients. Thirty-one grafts had an angiographically proven outflow stenosis. A single venous pressure measurement at a blood flow of 200ml/minute (VP 200) was higher, and graft flow lower, in patients with a stenosis compared to those without. Whilst VP 200 detected stenoses in the outflow tract, arterial inflow resistance was also found to be an important determinant of total graft resistance and therefore of blood flow. As a result, blood flow did not correlate with VP measurements, which missed stenoses elsewhere in the graft. No data were collected on which measurement was superior in predicting thrombosis, although the authors assume that graft blood flow dictates the likelihood of thrombosis. A meta-analysis, published in 1999, using data from eight studies concluded that a single measurement of blood flow did not have enough accuracy to be a clinically useful predictor of blood flow [7]. Critics have argued that neither a single measurement of blood flow rate nor a falling blood flow over sequential measurement is sufficiently predictive of incipient thrombosis, and that duplex ultrasound for detection of significant stenoses is also required for optimal selection of patients who should undergo angiography [4]. Although ultrasound dilution has now been endorsed by the US National Kidney Foundation Disease Outcomes Quality Initiative [25], there is still disagreement on how reliable the evidence is that this is the best technique for the detection of the access at risk of thrombosis. Clinical Practice Guidelines issued by the Renal Association recommend investigation of a fistula or graft for arterial or venous stenosis or access recirculation if there is a significant fall in the blood flow rate that can be achieved, a reduction in delivered dialysis dose, or a persistent rise in venous pressure in sequential dialysis sessions [26].

Conclusions

Any surveillance program which focuses the clinician's attention on the possibility of vascular access failure and increases the use of angiography with a view to angioplasty or surgical correction of severe stenosis is likely to result in a major improvement in thrombosis rates, independent of the methods used - if the default state is that of waiting for a thrombosis to

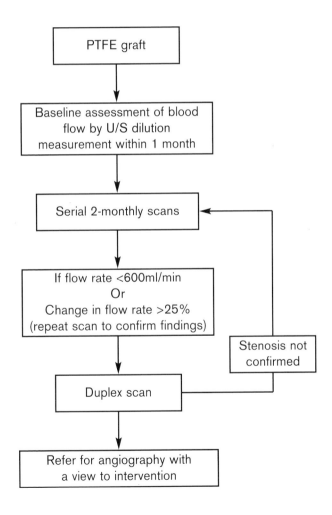

Figure 1 Flow diagram for PTFE graft surveillance.

occur before investigation. Despite conflicting evidence from studies it is likely that serial measurements of access blood flow by ultrasound dilution is a useful method of surveillance of PTFE grafts and most able to identify patients in need of further investigation. There is also some evidence that patients with autogenous AV fistulae may benefit from surveillance. Figure 1 summarises a possible regimen for surveillance of PTFE grafts using blood flow measurements. If a program of surveillance is to be set up, prompt access to interventional services is necessary. Further research should focus on the most cost-effective use of surveillance methodology. The role and cost-effectiveness of routine duplex ultrasonography in surveillance - as opposed to investigation of grafts with falling blood flow - remains to be defined by an adequately powered randomised controlled trial.

Key Summary

◆ Repeated measurement of blood flow using ultrasound dilution is currently regarded as the most cost-effective way of identifying PTFE grafts at risk of failure.

◆ There is increasing evidence to support the surveillance of autogenous AV fistulae.

◆ Duplex ultrasonography is the first choice investigation for the failing access and has a key role in selection of patients for radiological intervention.

◆ Further studies are required to define the optimum method and frequency of surveillance.

References

1. Garland JS, Moist LM, Lindsay RM. Are haemodialysis access flow measurements by ultrasound dilution the standard of care for access surveillance? *Adv Ren Replac Ther* 2002; 9: 91-8.

2. Harvey R, Bredenberg CE, Couper L, *et al.* Aspirin enhances platelet-derived growth factor-induced vascular smooth muscle cell proliferation. *J Vasc Surg* 1997; 25: 689-95.

3. Wetzig GA, Gough IR, Furnival CM. One hundred cases of arteriovenous fistula for haemodialysis access: the effect of cigarette smoking on patency. *ANZ J Surg* 1985; 55: 551-4.

4. Paulson WD. Blood flow surveillance of hemodialysis grafts and the dysfunction hypothesis. *Semin Dial* 2001; 14: 175-80.

5. Ronco C, Brendolan A, Crepaldi C, *et al.* Noninvasive transcutaneous access flow measurement before and after hemodialysis: impact of hematocrit and blood pressure. *Blood Purif* 2002; 20: 376-9.

6. Besarab A, Lubkowski T, Vu A, *et al.* Effects of systemic hemodynamics on flow within vascular accesses used for hemodialysis. *ASAIO J* 2001; 47: 501-6.

7. Paulson WD, Ram SJ, Birk CG, *et al.* Does blood flow accurately predict thrombosis or failure of hemodialysis synthetic grafts? A meta-analysis. *Am J Kidney Dis* 1999; 34: 478-85.

8. Kemp HJ, Parnham A, Tomson CR. Urea kinetic modelling: a measure of dialysis adequacy. *Ann Clin Biochem* 2001; 38: 20-7.

9. Schwab SJ, Raymond JR, Saeed M, *et al.* Prevention of hemodialysis fistula thrombosis. Early detection of venous stenoses. *Kidney Int* 1989; 36: 707-11.

10. Besarab A, Sullivan KL, Ross RP, *et al.* Utility of intra-access pressure monitoring in detecting and correcting venous outlet stenoses prior to thrombosis. *Kidney Int* 1995; 47: 1364-73.

11. McCarley P, Wingard RL, Shyr Y, *et al.* Vascular access blood flow monitoring reduces access morbidity and costs. *Kidney Int* 2001; 60: 1164-72.

12. Besarab A, Frinak S, Sherman RA, *et al.* Simplified measurement of intra-access pressure. *J Am Soc Nephrol* 1998; 9: 284-9.

13. Smits JH, van der Linden J, Hagen EC, *et al.* Graft surveillance: venous pressure, access flow, or the combination? *Kidney Int* 2001; 59: 1551-8.

14. Krivitski NM. Theory and validation of access flow measurement by dilution technique during hemodialysis. *Kidney Int* 1995; 48: 244-50.

15. Schwab SJ, Oliver MJ, Suhocki P, *et al.* Hemodialysis arteriovenous access: detection of stenosis and response to treatment by vascular access blood flow. *Kidney Int* 2001; 59: 358-62.

16. Tonelli M, Jindal K, Hirsch D, *et al.* Screening for subclinical stenosis in native vessel arteriovenous fistulae. *J Am Soc Nephrol* 2001; 12: 1729-33.

17. May RE, Himmelfarb J, Yenicesu M, *et al.* Predictive measures of vascular access thrombosis: a prospective study. *Kidney Int* 1997; 52: 1656-62.

18. Zanen AL, Toonder IM, Korten E, *et al.* Flow measurements in dialysis shunts: lack of agreement between conventional Doppler, CVI-Q, and ultrasound dilution. *Nephrol Dial Transplant* 2001; 16: 395-9.

19. Gadallah MF, Paulson WD, Vickers B, *et al.* Accuracy of Doppler ultrasound in diagnosing anatomic stenosis of hemodialysis arteriovenous access as compared with fistulography. *Am J Kid Dis* 1998; 32: 273-7.

20. Bosman PJ, Boereboom FT, Smits HF, *et al.* Pressure or flow recordings for the surveillance of haemodialysis grafts. *Kidney Int* 1997; 52: 1084-8.

21. Tessitore N, Lipari G, Poli A, *et al.* Can blood flow surveillance and pre-emptive repair of subclinical stenosis prolong the useful life of arteriovenous fistulae? A randomised controlled study. *Nephrol Dial Transplant* 2004; 19: 2325-33.

22. Sands JJ, Jabyac PJ, Miranda CL, *et al.* Intervention based on monthly monitoring decreases haemodialysis access thrombosis. *ASAIO J* 1999; 45: 147-50.

23. Besarab A. Access monitoring is worthwhile and valuable. *Blood Purif* 2006; 24: 77-89.

24. Treacy PJ, Ragg JL, Snelling P, *et al.* Prediction of native arteriovenous fistulas using 'on-line' fistula flow measurements. *Nephrology* (Carlton) 2005; 10: 136-41.

25. National Kidney Foundation Kidney Disease Outcomes Quality Initiative, 2006. http://www.kidney.org/professionals/kdoqi/guideline_upHD_PD_VA/va_guide4.htm.

26. Mactier M, Davies S. Clinical Practice Guidelines for Haemodialysis. UK Renal Association, 4th Edition, 2006. Available on www.renal.org.

Chapter 13

Interventions to restore or maintain access patency

Peter WG Brown BSc FRCS FRCR

Consultant Radiologist, Sheffield Teaching Hospitals NHS Trust, Sheffield, UK

Introduction

Access dysfunction is a leading cause of hospital admission for patients undergoing haemodialysis. Native arteriovenous (AV) fistulae are common in Europe and offer the most durable type of access with patency rates at one year of 75-91%. Prosthetic grafts are less reliable with one-year patency rates of around 55%. Until recently they were the preferred option in the US, but now, native fistulae are increasingly common. Prompt investigation and treatment of a failing access is a priority, as delay may lead to thrombosis, which can be difficult to treat and is associated with poor long-term patency. Most reports of the treatment of access dysfunction are from the US, partly due to the high prevalence of synthetic grafts, which need more frequent intervention. There is less information on the management of native AV fistulae, mostly from Europe.

The traditional therapy for a failing haemodialysis access has been surgical thrombectomy with or without revision. Over the last 20 years the advantages of an endovascular approach have become clear with minimal invasion, better imaging and improved venous preservation. Balloon angioplasty with or without stenting is now routinely used to maintain access patency and a variety of techniques have evolved to declot thrombosed fistulae. Thrombolysis, pharmacomechancial thrombolysis and mechanical thrombectomy each have their advocates and specific uses. The wide variety of declotting techniques described suggests that none is optimal. There is also limited literature comparing surgical thrombectomy with endovascular techniques and the optimum management of the thrombosed fistula has yet to be defined.

In the UK the haemodialysis population is expanding approximately at 8% per year but limited resources compromise the management of failing fistulae. There are shortages of interventional radiologists and vascular access surgeons, and centres have widely different practices. The American DOQI (Dialysis Outcomes Quality Initiative) guidelines [1] and standards of practice guidelines of the Society of Cardiovascular and Interventional Radiology [2] have defined best practice but have had little impact in the UK, where radiological or surgical interventions often depend on local resources and expertise.

Indications for intervention

There is good evidence that elective intervention to treat haemodynamically significant stenoses (>50% reduction of normal vessel diameter with a haemodynamic, functional or clinical abnormality) reduces the rate of thrombosis and graft loss, and prolongs the life of an access (DOQI guideline 17). Thrombosis is roughly ten times more frequent in prosthetic grafts than native fistulae. It is essential to establish the cause and an underlying venous stenosis is unmasked in over 90% of grafts and most native fistulae. Venous stenoses are commonly found in the peri-anastomotic region of native fistulae and venous outflow of grafts (Figure 1).

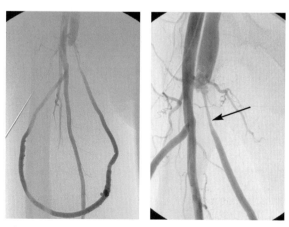

Figure 1 A typical outflow stenosis (arrow) at the venous end of a thigh PTFE loop graft.

If an underlying stenosis of a thrombosed graft is not corrected, there is at least a 90% chance of rapid rethrombosis.

Stenosis detection

There is increasing evidence that the patency of vascular access grafts can be extended by regular monitoring and early intervention. The evidence for surveillance of native fistulae is less strong.

Early signs of access dysfunction can be detected by serial in-line access flow measurements or elevated static and dynamic venous pressures. Dialysis centres should have strict screening protocols, ideally based on flow measurements, but comprehensive screening is rare in the UK. Patients are usually referred to an access surgeon when there are increasing venous pressures, poor pump speeds or needling problems. Ideally, a multidisciplinary team should assess patients, including an access surgeon, an interventional radiologist, a nephrologist and a dialysis nurse. Technical difficulties with dialysis can be discussed and appropriate investigations and intervention planned.

Careful clinical examination remains the key to accurate assessment. Stenoses can sometimes be directly palpated and other useful signs include localised loss or reinforcement of thrill, venous hypertension and aneurysm formation. In many patients imaging is unnecessary and appropriate intervention, whether surgical or radiological, can be planned after clinical assessment alone. Others will require duplex ultrasound or fistulography to clarify the cause of the access dysfunction.

Angioplasty

Technique

Duplex ultrasound is useful for planning fistulography and access for intervention, and is ideally performed in the angiography room. Stenoses can easily be visualised and an appropriate puncture site can be chosen for optimal access (Figure 2).

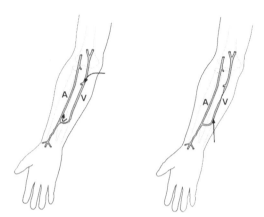

Figure 2 The forearm cephalic vein is accessed for fistulography with a view to angioplasty, either proximally or distally depending on the location of the venous stenosis.

Pre-dilatation fistulography is usually performed by puncturing the graft or vein, reserving puncture of the brachial artery for the diagnosis of inflow problems. The brachial route has also been advocated for angioplasty access [3], but should be generally discouraged because of a higher rate of puncture site complications. An initial contrast injection should be performed with a proximal blood pressure cuff inflated above arterial pressure, to allow satisfactory visualisation of the arterial anastomosis and inflow artery. It is also important to visualise fully the venous run-off from the fistula and the subclavian and central veins to exclude stenoses.

Most angioplasties can be performed through a 5 or 6 French (Fr.) sheath. A radio-opaque tip is particularly useful to orientate the sheath near the stenosis. Stenoses are usually crossed with a hydrophilic wire before exchanging for a standard wire over which the angioplasty is performed (Figure 3).

Most radiologists administer 3000 to 5000 units of heparin during the procedure. Although venous stenoses can be very difficult to dilate, an initial attempt with a standard angioplasty balloon (pressure up to 15 atmospheres) is often successful. Balloon inflation can be very painful and local infiltration of anaesthetic or sedation is necessary. Most authors

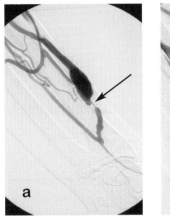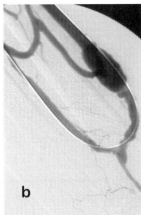

Figure 3 a) A typical tight peri-anastomotic stenosis (arrow) in an autogenous forearm fistula. b) This responds well to angioplasty.

suggest that slight over-dilatation gives the best results. For the venous anastomosis of a 6mm graft a 6-8mm balloon should be used. There is little consensus regarding balloon inflation time. In the Netherlands, prolonged inflation times with a distal perfusion balloon are advocated but most radiologists dilate for 1-2 minutes after abolishing the waist on the balloon. Arterial inflow stenoses are uncommon and are best dilated with arterial access using standard techniques.

Resistant stenoses

Some venous stenoses are particularly resistant to dilatation. A recent study has shown that 55% of overall lesions require pressures greater than 15 atmospheres to efface the waist on the angioplasty balloon, with 20% of native fistulae requiring more than 20 atmospheres. The cutting balloon, with several tiny blades attached, is often successful but the incidence of venous rupture is greater and such balloons are relatively expensive. Patency rates six months after angioplasty with cutting and standard balloons are similar [4].

An alternative is ultra-high-pressure angioplasty balloons that can be inflated up to 40 atmospheres. These are effective at treating nearly all resistant stenoses and are less expensive than cutting balloons. It has been suggested that cutting balloons should be a last resort after high-pressure balloons have failed (less than 2% of procedures).

Complications

Angioplasty of stenosed dialysis fistulae is relatively safe. Morbidity rates of 2-15% have been reported including iodine allergies, infection, thrombosis and vessel rupture. Venous ruptures occur in about 1.7% of cases and can be relatively easily treated by self-expanding stents. Small ruptures can often be controlled by prolonged low-pressure balloon inflations.

Results

Technical success for angioplasty of stenosed grafts and AV fistulae (defined as less than 30% residual stenosis and resumption of normal dialysis) of over 90% is generally expected. However, restenosis is a major problem for both grafts and native fistulae.

Grafts

Most large studies report primary patencies of around 60% at six months and 30% at one year. Secondary patency at one year can be as high as 90%.

Autogenous fistulae

Primary patency rates for forearm fistulae at six months and one year are similar to those of grafts in most reports, but a small UK series reported better results for fistulae of 77% patency at six months and 64% at one year. Secondary patency rates of more than 80% at one year were reported from a large French series but upper arm fistulae needed more frequent intervention. Similarly, grafts need more frequent interventions than fistulae to achieve high secondary patency rates.

Other prognostic factors
Other prognostic factors are:

◆   previous thrombosis reduces patency after angioplasty;
◆   occlusions and lesions longer than 6cm have reduced technical success and patency;
◆   access age - the older the fistula at the time of angioplasty, the better the results;
◆   anastomotic stenoses are associated with poor results;
◆   small size of the feeding artery is associated with poor results.

Central venous stenosis

Central vein stenoses and occlusions are usually caused by previous central vein catheterisation (Figure 4).

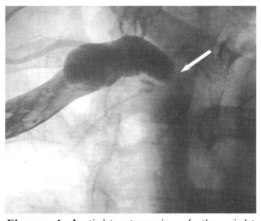

Figure 4 A tight stenosis of the right subclavian vein origin due to a previous central venous catheter.

The results of simple angioplasty are poor, with 23-29% primary patency rates at six months. Central venous stenoses frequently show elastic recoil after dilatation, which may be an indication for stent placement. Nevertheless, successful angioplasty, even if associated with some elastic recoil, can dramatically improve limb oedema, albeit for a limited time. As central vein stenoses are difficult to treat and have limited long-term patency, consideration should be given to the insertion of a further fistula in another limb, if this is possible.

Intragraft stenosis

Intragraft stenoses occur in approximately 30% of patients with failing access. Balloon angioplasty is effective and has similar patency rates to directional and pullback atherectomy.

Immature fistulae

AV fistula development depends on an inflow adequate to support effective dialysis and sufficient venous maturation to allow repeated cannulation with a 15-16 G needle. Small or atherosclerotic arteries can cause primary non-function. Venous maturation may be delayed with veins smaller than 2.5mm, the development of venous stenoses, or by diversion of blood flow via large accessory veins. Some fistulae may be difficult to needle because the draining vein lies deep. Venous stenoses associated with immature fistulae respond well to dilatation. Opinion is divided as to whether side branch ligation speeds up maturation.

Comparison with surgery

In forearm fistulae surgery gives slightly better one-year primary patencies (65-84%) than angioplasty (51%). If angioplasty is used, early surgical revision should be considered if there is rapid restenosis. In other native fistulae and grafts, angioplasty is preferred as it preserves veins for further access. Surgery is recommended in all groups if more than two angioplasties are required in a three-month interval to maintain patency (DOQI guideline 19).

Stents

Stents can be useful in some circumstances but are prone to recurrent stenosis within or adjacent to the stent. They are particularly useful for rupture control following failure of prolonged balloon inflation, and for significant stenosis recoil. The stent should be self-expanding and 1-2mm greater than the largest balloon size.

Three American randomised trials showed no benefit of stent placement over balloon angioplasty for the treatment of venous outflow stenoses of PTFE grafts, with similar patencies at six and 12 months. In contrast, non-randomised retrospective studies suggest that selective stenting may delay restenosis and decrease the frequency of necessary intervention. Indications for stent placement would be stenosis recoil, acute rupture and early stenosis recurrence. It has been suggested that the poor results from the randomised studies could be due to balloon under-dilatation before stent placement.

There is some evidence from Germany that stents are effective as a primary treatment for central vein stenosis, reporting primary patencies at one year of up to 70%, although studies from the US described six-month and one-year patencies of only 42% and 25%. Secondary patency may be much higher with repeated intervention. Even the poor American results are better than intervention with angioplasty alone and most authors would agree that central veins should be stented if there is significant recoil after angioplasty.

Important technical points in placing a central venous stent are [5]:

◆ a stent placed in the subclavian vein must not overlap the origin of a patent internal jugular vein and compromise future catheter access;
◆ a stent placed in either brachiocephalic vein must not protrude into the superior vena cava. This may compromise future catheter access through the contralateral brachiocephalic vein and induce a stenosis (Figure 5);

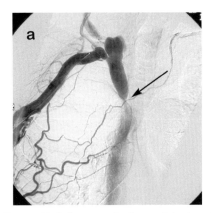 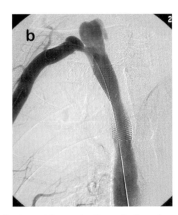

Figure 5 a) A stenosis (arrow) in the right brachiocephalic vein has been treated by the insertion of a stent. b) The stent almost certainly overlaps the left brachiocephalic vein origin compromising all future catheter access from the left side.

◆ a stent placed in the final arch of the cephalic vein must not protrude into and compromise the adjacent subclavian vein.

These important technical points often preclude stent placement. A stent placed at the subclavian vein origin may also be traumatised in the relatively small space between the first rib and clavicle.

Declotting

The traditional treatment of a thrombosed access is surgical thrombectomy. Thrombectomy alone has poor results without revision or dilatation of any underlying venous stenosis. Percutaneous techniques have advantages over surgery as they allow accurate treatment with balloon angioplasty (+/- stenting) and are less invasive. A large variety of endovascular techniques have been recently developed to allow rapid clot removal with minimal complications. Most work has been performed in grafts, which are more prone to thrombosis than native AV fistulae. The fact that so many different methods have been reported suggests that no single technique is optimal.

Principles

The principles of declotting are:

◆ the venous outflow stenosis must be treated adequately. This determines the success and patency of the intervention;

◆ the percutaneous approach must allow access to all parts of the fistula/graft. This intervention usually means crossed catheters or an apex puncture in grafts;

◆ the arterial plug must be adequately treated. This is a lysis-resistant organised plug found at the arterial end of the thrombosed grafts and native fistulae. It consists of compressed laminated layers of erythrocytes and fibrin;

◆ whichever declotting method is used, it must be readily available, rapidly effective, cheap and with few complications;

◆ venous outflow stenoses should be negotiated and the patency of central veins assessed before declotting. There is no point proceeding without establishing an outflow.

Early percutaneous attempts to declot grafts used a prolonged infusion of thrombolytic (streptokinase or urokinase), through a needle or short catheter. Whilst some interventions were successful, there were high failure rates, long infusion times and a significant number of bleeding complications. Frustration with pharmacologic infusions led early investigators to turn to mechanical techniques to assist traditional thrombolysis. Initially this was with external massage, but later forceful injections of thrombolytic through catheters with multiple side holes were used (the pulse spray technique). These pharmaco-mechanical methods were often supplemented with angioplasty of residual clot, and this led to the development of pure mechanical declotting techniques such as hydrodynamic thrombectomy, mechanical fragmentation and thrombus aspiration. The exact method of declotting is not important provided it is readily available and there is local expertise. It is treatment of residual clot and the venous outflow stenosis, which affect long-term patency.

Current techniques

Pharmacological thrombolysis

Techniques based primarily on thrombolysis, which can be used in grafts include:

◆   high-dose infusion: a lytic agent in high concentration (e.g urokinase) is infused through crossed catheters over approximately one hour;
◆   'lyse and wait': a mixture of heparin (5000 units) and urokinase (250,000 units) in a volume of 10ml is slowly infused into the graft over one minute through a 22G catheter pointing towards the venous anastomosis. The infusion is performed on the ward before the patient is transferred to angiography 30 minutes to two hours later. A variation on this technique is 'lyse and go' in which the graft is quickly accessed after the infusion and treated by supplemental mechanical techniques. Great care must be taken to avoid arterial embolisation during any infusion into a thrombosed graft.

With both techniques mobilisation and angioplasty of the arterial plug is usually necessary to re-establish flow, as well as angioplasty of the usual outflow stenosis.

Thrombolysis is occasionally useful in native fistulae with a small amount of thrombus, particularly if there is extension into the feeding artery. Most radiologists lace the clot with a small dose of tissue plasminogen activator (2-4mg).

Pharmaco-mechanical thrombolysis

'Pulse spray thrombolysis' allows greater surface area of clot to be exposed to thrombolytic agent compared to conventional lacing and is usually supplemented with external massage, balloon maceration and aggressive treatment of the arterial plug. Two catheters with multiple side-holes and tip occluding wires are placed in a crisscross fashion in the thrombosed graft (Figure 6).

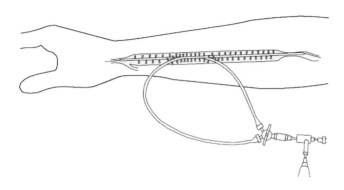

Figure 6 'Pulsed spray thrombolysis'. Two crossed catheters are inserted into a thrombosed graft, which is thrombolysed by forceful injection of thrombolytic agent.

Forceful and rapid injections of 0.2-0.3ml aliquots of a 10ml mixture combining 250,000ml of urokinase and 5000 units of heparin are applied every 30 seconds in each catheter with a tuberculin syringe. Pulsed spray techniques are faster, more successful, and safer than pure pharmacologic techniques. Serious complications (bleeding, angioplasty rupture, peripheral and symptomatic central emboli) occur in about 1% of cases.

Mechanical techniques
Mechanical techniques have recently become popular for treating thrombosed AV fistulae. The large number described suggests that no single technique is yet optimal:

◆ pulsed spray with heparinised saline and balloon maceration: this has been shown to be as effective as pulsed spray with urokinase but may have a higher rate of pulmonary embolism [6];

◆ aspiration thrombectomy: clot removal can be performed with a simple 7 or 8 Fr. aspiration catheter. The angled catheter is slowly withdrawn and rotated through the thrombus whilst aspirating with a

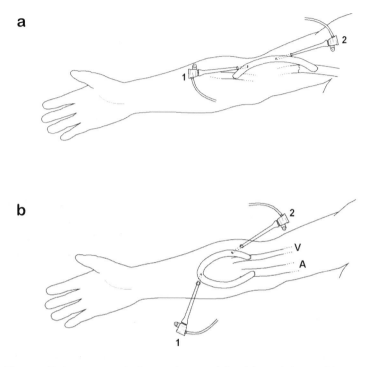

Figure 7 Access techniques for straight (a) and loop (b) grafts. The venous sheath (1) is placed before the arterial sheath (2). The sheaths must not overlap.

50ml syringe. This technique is simple and cost effective but requires considerable expertise;

◆ hydrodynamic thrombectomy: three different devices are commonly used: the Hydrolyser (Cordis, Roden Netherlands), the Oasis catheter (Boston Scientific, Natich, Mass, USA) and the Angiojet catheter (Possis Inc, USA). All work using the same principle. They are double-lumen catheters with a retrograde saline injection from a small supply lumen that is injected at high pressure into a larger efferent lumen. This creates a hydrodynamic vortex (Venturi effect), fragmenting surrounding thrombus before it is sucked into the exhaust lumen mixed with saline;

◆ endoluminal clot dissolution: this technique causes mechanical fragmentation of thrombus, which is then aspirated or deliberately embolised. Specific devices which are available are: the Amplatz thrombectomy device (Microvena, Minneapolis, USA), the Arrow Trerotola Thrombectomy Device (Arrow Inc, USA), the minipigtail catheter (Cook Europe, Bjaeverskov, Denmark), and the Cragg Thrombolytic Brush Catheter (TBC Microtherapeutics, Irvine, California, USA). There is some evidence that these are more effective at removing adherent wall thrombus than other mechanical devices.

Access for mechanical devices in both fistulae and grafts is generally in a crossed catheter approach (Figure 7). The sheaths must not overlap or complete thrombus removal will not be possible. The venous sheath is normally placed first. This allows venography to confirm patency of the venous drainage and accesses the usual outflow stenosis.

The arterial plug

The arterial plug tends to be difficult to remove either with thrombolysis or mechanical devices. Usually the best way to dislodge the plug is by balloon thrombectomy using a Fogarty balloon catheter. The catheter is placed beyond the plug and the balloon inflated. The balloon is pulled back against the plug, forcing it into the graft where it can be crushed or embolised into the venous circulation.

Residual thrombus and the venous stenosis

With all declotting techniques there is usually residual clot in the graft or native fistula following restoration of flow. It is essential to clear this as much as possible to prevent early rethrombosis. Usually residual thrombosis can be crushed with a balloon or deliberately embolised to the lungs. Once the access is running it is essential to check the underlying cause of the thrombosis has been adequately treated before sheath removal.

In patients with grafts a simple 2/0 purse string suture can be placed around the sheath before removal to facilitate haemostasis. The suture passes through perigraft fibrosis but not the graft itself and is very effective at controlling bleeding without compromising the graft.

Complications

The most dangerous complication of declotting is embolisation either directly to the lungs or into the systemic arterial tree via a patent foramen ovale or right to left shunt. Despite this, only six deaths directly linked to the procedure have been reported. Other significant complications include arterial embolisation (1-9%), vessel rupture (2-3%) and bleeding (2-3%).

All methods of declotting and particular mechanical techniques cause central displacement of thrombus. This is nearly always asymptomatic as the overall total volume of thrombus in a graft is only about 3ml. There has been concern that some embolisation, even of small amounts of clot, could be dangerous in dialysis patients with a cardiopulmonary disease and repeated declotting procedures over time may cause pulmonary hypertension [7]. In practice the risk of a life-threatening pulmonary embolus is very small. Particular care must be taken to reduce the risk of embolisation in high-risk patients with pulmonary hypertension, e.g. clot dissolution techniques.

Results

Grafts

Clinical success rates (the ability to perform at least one full dialysis treatment through the clotted graft) of graft declotting with all current techniques range from 72% to 100%. It is probably not important which technique is used, but it is essential that an experienced radiologist carries out the procedure and that it can be quickly arranged. Primary patency rates at one month (32-84%) depend more on complete thrombus removal and how the underlying stenosis is treated, rather than the particular declotting technique. These procedures usually take 60 to 120 minutes. Long-term primary patencies are poor ranging from 8-26% at one year. Secondary patency rates are more encouraging reaching 75% at one year.

Autogenous fistulae

Techniques include thrombolysis and angioplasty, thrombo-aspiration and the use of several mechanical devices (Arrow Trerotola PTD, Hydrolyser, Amplatz thrombectomy device and minipigtail). Clinical success rates of up to 100% have been reported. Specific difficulties encountered with native fistulae include extensive thrombus in aneurysmal veins and long venous stenoses or occlusions. Primary patency rates at one year range from 9% to 49% with higher patencies in forearm fistulae than upper arm fistulae. High secondary patency rates of up to 81% are reported with repeated intervention.

Comparison with surgical techniques

There have been few direct comparisons of endovascular and surgical techniques in access declotting. Both thrombolytic and mechanical techniques have been compared but the results are controversial. Surgical and endovascular techniques appear to have similar technical success and long-term patency. Endovascular techniques are less invasive and allow venous preservation. However, surgical declotting, if combined with revision of the native fistula or graft venous anastomosis, probably has a better long-term patency than endovascular intervention, but this remains to be proven by randomised trials. The choice of surgical or radiological declotting usually depends on local circumstances, individual patient-related factors and available expertise.

Conclusions

Endovascular techniques are essential for the optimum management of failing AV fistulae and grafts. Angioplasty is a safe and effective technique but may need to be repeated to achieve satisfactory patency rates. Stenting should be considered in the treatment of central vein stenosis. There are a wide variety of declotting techniques and all require treatment of the underlying stenosis and removal of residual clot to be effective. Failing AV fistulae and grafts should be managed by a multidisciplinary team.

Key Summary

◆ Prosthetic grafts thrombose more often than autogenous fistulae and require more frequent intervention to maintain patency.

◆ Venous stenoses are commonly found in the peri-anastomotic region of native fistulae and venous outflow of grafts.

◆ Elective intervention on failing fistulae with angioplasty is safe and effective at preventing thrombosis but frequent procedures are required to achieve satisfactory long-term patency.

◆ Indications for stents are limited. They are probably of value in central vein stenoses if carefully placed.

◆ There is no consensus about the best technique to declot a thrombosed access. It is essential to adequately treat the underlying stenosis to achieve satisfactory long-term patency.

◆ All declotting techniques cause pulmonary emboli. These may be significant in patients undergoing multiple procedures or with pulmonary hypertension.

◆ Optimum management of failing fistulae is often determined by local expertise and resources, and should be via a multidisciplinary approach.

References

1.　Schwab S, Besarab A, Beathard G, *et al*. NKF-DOQI clinical practice guidelines for vascular access. *Am J Kidney Disease* 1977; 30: Suppl 4.

2.　Aruny J, Lewis C, Cardella J, *et al*. Quality improvement guidelines for percutaneous management of the thrombosed or dysfunctional dialysis access. *J Vasc Interv Radiol* 1999; 10: 491-8.

3.　Manninen H, Kaukanen E, Ikaheimo R, *et al*. Brachial arterial access: endovascular treatment of failing Brescia-Cimino haemodialysis fistulae - initial success and long-term results. *Radiology* 2001; 218: 711-8.

4.　Vessely TM, Siegel JB. Use of the cutting balloon to treat hemodialysis-related stenoses. *J Vasc Interv Radiol* 2005; 16: 1593-603.

5.　Turmel-Rodrigues L, Pengloan J, Bourquelot P. Interventional radiology in haemodialysis fistulae and grafts: a multidisciplinary approach. *Cardiovasc Intervent Radiol* 2002; 25: 3-16.

6.　Beathard G. Mechanical thrombolysis for the treatment of thrombosed haemodialysis access grafts. *Radiology* 1996; 200: 711-6.

7.　Dolmatch B, Gray R, Horton K. Will iatrogenic pulmonary embolism be our pulmonary embarrassment? *Radiology* 1994; 191: 615-7.

Chapter 14

Why peritoneal dialysis?

Edwina Brown DM FRCP

Consultant Nephrologist, West London Renal and Transplant Centre

Hammersmith Hospital, London, UK

Introduction

The aims of renal replacement therapy (RRT) are not simply correction of blood abnormalities and maintenance of fluid balance. Patients can live on renal replacement treatment for decades so that the aim is for them to live as normal a life as possible. It is therefore important that they utilise a mode of RRT that they tolerate well, and therefore comply with, that provides physical well-being, and allows social and employment rehabilitation. Although a randomised study has not been done (and never will be), evidence from various national registries shows that overall, patient survival is the same whether patients start on haemodialysis (HD) or peritoneal dialysis (PD) [1].

For patients who can use any modality, the choice of HD or PD will depend on individual patient preference, nephrologist bias and local resources. In the UK, around 26.5% of new patients start on PD, although 80% of patients over the age of 65 years are on HD at 90 days, compared with 64.3% of patients less than 65 years old [2]. The principal advantages of PD are that it is a home-based treatment, vascular access is not required, there is less cardiovascular stress in patients with poor cardiac function, and quality of life may be better for many older patients. The relative advantages and disadvantages of HD and PD are shown in Table 1.

Table 1 Comparison of haemodialysis and peritoneal dialysis.

	Haemodialysis	Peritoneal dialysis
Dialysis procedure	• Mostly dependent on nurses and technicians • Session times dependent on availability in unit and can be at antisocial hours • Independent of patient's ability to learn or carry out technique	• Carried out by patient in own home • Dialysis can be fitted round patient's lifestyle • Dependent on patient or family member performing technique
Travel	• Arrangements need to be made with a local HD unit prior to travel • Patient has to dialyse at times offered by unit	• PD fluid can be delivered to most parts of world with prior notice
Access for dialysis	• Need to allow 2 - 3 months for fistula before useable • Fistulae can be difficult to create in diabetics or patients with arterial disease • Acute access with central venous catheters have a high complication rate: infection, thrombosis, venous stenosis	• Access easy to establish • PD catheter can be used immediately, but advisable to allow to heal for 2 weeks
Infection complications	• Septicaemia associated with catheter infections can be life-threatening • Complications of catheter infections often dangerous, e.g. subacute bacterial endocarditis, septic arthritis, epidural abscess	• Catheter exit-site infection - rarely serious • Peritonitis - if serious, usually resolves after catheter removal; rarely fatal
Cardiovascular complications	• Risk of hypotension with fluid removal - increased if poor cardiac function • Arrhythmias can occur as plasma potassium falls during dialysis • Angina, myocardial infarction and stroke can be precipitated by hypotensive episode	• Fluid overload can occur if poor ultrafiltration • Safer for patients with poor cardiac function, severe ischaemic heart disease or cerebrovascular disease

Table 1 *Continued*:

	Haemodialysis	Peritoneal dialysis
Psychosocial	• Not suitable for patients with needle phobia • Body image problems with fistula, particularly young women • Can be inconvenient for family or social support as patient may have to dialyse at antisocial hours and require help with transport	• Body image problems with PD catheter - may prevent patient from accepting PD • Dependent on patient or family member being able to learn and comply with technique • 'Burnout' - occurs after long period of time on PD • Care of dependent family member can be easier if dialysis carried out at home and life not disrupted by 3/week hospital visits
Contraindications	• Inability to achieve vascular access • Severe ischaemic heart disease • Severe heart failure	• Presence of colostomy, ileostomy or ileal conduit • Intra-abdominal adhesions • Inoperable hernia
Survival	• Survival on PD and HD similar for first 3 - 4 years • High technique survival - low dropout to PD because of lack of vascular access • Experience with long-term patient survival for 20 years plus	• Survival on PD and HD similar for first 3 - 4 years • Relatively high dropout rate because of peritonitis, poor ultrafiltration, or inadequate dialysis when residual renal function lost • Increasing risk of encapsulating peritoneal sclerosis after 5 years

PD as a home dialysis treatment

Many patients prefer the independence of home dialysis, as this enables them to take control of their own treatment, increases their ability to fit treatment round work schedules and family commitments and, with PD, makes travel easier. PD is technically much easier than home haemodialysis and is therefore usually the modality chosen by patients who would prefer a home treatment when starting dialysis. Dialysing at home avoids the need for regular transport to and from the dialysis unit. This is one of the principal areas of complaint of any group of HD patients and can easily extend a four-hour treatment to occupy the whole day, often at anti-social hours, particularly for patients dependent on hospital-provided transport.

Preservation of vascular access

Achieving successful vascular access remains the Achilles heel of haemodialysis. The possibility of switching to PD should therefore be discussed with patients who are having difficulties with their vascular access or who no longer have potential vascular access sites, either for fistula creation, or central line insertion. The European APD Outcome Study [3] included many patients who had switched to PD because of vascular access problems and showed that the survival of anuric patients on PD was similar to survival rates on HD. Starting new patients on PD avoids the need to use vascular access in the early stages of life with end-stage kidney disease. Vascular access sites can then be preserved until some time later when PD has failed; in patients having a transplant, this can be many years later. The use of PD in this way has led to the concept of integrated care [4], whereby use of each treatment modality (PD, HD, transplantation) are made available to all patients and used at appropriate times with changes in therapy being anticipated and accepted, and not being seen as a mark of treatment failure.

Choice of dialysis modality for older patients

The median age of starting on dialysis in the UK is now around 65 years [2]. Older patients with end-stage kidney disease often have considerable comorbidity, not only the vascular problems associated with their renal disease, but also the comorbidity found in all elderly people, namely impaired vision, deafness, poor mobility, arthritis and cognitive problems. They are often socially isolated, may well have financial problems and are often depressed due to loss of independence or bereavement. These factors are all problematic for any dialysis modality. For HD, the associated vascular disease results in a high risk of failure for vascular access. This results in increased reliance on venous access with all the associated risks of infection. Failure of vascular access can necessitate frequent hospital admissions for often unpleasant and painful radiological and surgical procedures. Cardiac disease in these patients can also cause hypotension and arrythmias while on HD. Elderly patients often therefore feel 'washed out' after a dialysis. Added to this is the need for patients to travel to and from the dialysis unit; many cannot do this independently and therefore require transport provided by the hospital. Not only may some have to travel long distances, but also there are frequently long waits for the transport that is often at antisocial times of the day.

PD has the advantage that it is done in the home thereby avoiding the need for transport. This is an advantage for both the fit and the more frail elderly. For the fit elderly, it means that they can travel, have an active social life and enjoy their retirement. The more frail elderly will generally feel better as they will not have the swings of HD and they will avoid the need for travel to the HD unit. The problem is to determine whether such individuals can cope with the rigours of a home treatment. Healthcare professionals often make the decision that PD is not an option without full discussion with the patient. Many older patients can be trained to do their own PD, although this may take longer than with younger patients. Family members are often willing to help with all or part of the procedure and in some parts of Europe, the use of community nurses enables elderly patients to be on PD in their own homes. Indeed, in France, PD is predominantly used by the elderly with a median age of starting PD of 71 years, and 21.5% over 80 years of age; about half of these patients have assistance from community nurses [5].

Quality of life on PD

PD enables patient independence. This is appreciated by many patients, not only those who work and travel, but also those who just do not like hospitals and keeping to rigid timetables. Evidence suggests that patients who chose PD do so because it allows increased autonomy and control [6]; further questioning of these patients showed that specific reasons for selecting PD included a preference to do dialysis in the home, flexibility of the schedule, ease of work, preference for doing dialysis alone, and ease of travel. Studies from the same investigators have also shown that PD patients in general are more satisfied with their overall care and believe that their treatment has less impact on their lives than HD patients [7].

Conclusions

All patients with end-stage kidney disease should have the opportunity to discuss all the various treatment options. Choosing one option does not preclude changing to another at the appropriate time. PD will be chosen by those patients wanting a home-based treatment, independence from hospital care and / or have poor or no vascular access for haemodialysis.

Key Summary

◆ Patients starting on dialysis should be informed about the different dialysis modalities available, thereby enabling them to choose the one most appropriate for their lifestyle.

◆ PD is a home-based treatment. The dialysis schedule is therefore more flexible than HD, thereby enabling patients to continue working and to travel. Families or carers can carry out the PD for older patients who can then be treated in their own homes and avoid the rigours of regular transport to and from hospital.

◆ Vascular access is not needed. By starting on PD, vascular access is preserved for later on in the patient pathway with end-stage kidney disease. PD should also be considered as an option for patients on HD who are struggling with their vascular access.

References

1. Vonesh EF, Snyder JJ, Foley RN, Collins AJ. Mortality studies comparing peritoneal dialysis and hemodialysis: what do they tell us? *Kidney Int* 2006; 70: S3-S11.

2. UK Renal Registry Report, 2005. UK Renal Registry, Bristol, UK.

3. Brown EA, Davies SJ, Rutherford P, *et al,* on behalf of EAPOS group. Survival of functionally anuric patients on Automated Peritoneal Dialysis: the European APD Outcome Study (EAPOS). *J Am Soc Nephrol* 2003; 14: 2948-57.

4. Davies SJ, van Biesen W, Nicholas J, Lameire N. Integrated care. *Perit Dial Int* 2001; 21 Suppl e: S269-74.

5. Verger C, Ryckelynck JP, Duman M, *et al.* French peritoneal dialysis registry (RDPLF): outline and main results. *Kidney Int* 2006; 70: S12-S20.

6. Wuerth DB, Finkelstein SH, Schwetz O, *et al.* Patients' descriptions of specific factors leading to modality selection of chronic peritoneal dialysis or haemodialysis. *Perit Dial Int* 2002; 22: 184-90.

7. Juergensen E, Wuerth D, Finkelstein SH, *et al.* Hemodialysis and peritoneal dialysis: patients' assessment of their satisfaction with therapy and the impact of the therapy on their lives. *Clin J Am Soc Nephrol* 2006; 1: 1191-6.

Chapter 15

Surgical aspects of peritoneal access

Badri M Shrestha BSc MS MPhil FRCS, *Consultant Surgeon*
Andrew T Raftery BSc MD FRCS, *Consultant Surgeon*
Sheffield Kidney Institute, Northern General Hospital, Sheffield, UK

Introduction

Peritoneal dialysis (PD) is preferred in motivated patients who are keen on PD and those with severe cardiac, extensive peripheral and central venous and arterial occlusive diseases. The provision of a safe, reliable, permanent and trouble-free access to the peritoneal cavity is vital to the patients on continuous ambulatory peritoneal dialysis (CAPD). There are numerous catheter designs and implantation techniques. The more common ones will be described in this chapter together with the pre-implantation preparation, contraindications to CAPD, surgical techniques of insertion of PD catheters, the complications of CAPD, the management of patients with abdominal problems who are already established on CAPD, and the management of CAPD catheters around the time of kidney transplantation.

Design of catheters

A variety of catheters is available for chronic peritoneal access. The standard, double cuff, straight Tenckhoff catheter is still the most widely used access device and there is no conclusive evidence that any other catheter is superior. Each catheter can be considered to consist of three segments [1]: extra-abdominal, intramural and intraperitoneal (Figure 1).

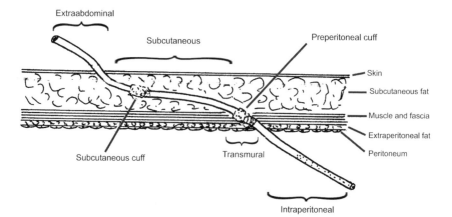

Figure 1 The parts of a peritoneal dialysis catheter.

Extra-abdominal

This is the part of the catheter, which protrudes from the exit site. It should be at least 10cm long for ease of handling. There should be enough length in reserve to allow trimming if a split occurs at the connection site to the giving set.

Intramural

This part of the catheter is contained within the abdominal wall tunnel which consists of transmural and subcutaneous segments. The transmural segment is the shortest section passing through the linea alba or abdominal wall muscles before entering the peritoneal cavity. It has three functions, i.e. the provision of mechanical anchorage, a water-tight peritoneal seal, and an antibacterial seal. This section should be designed and implanted to prevent catheter extrusion, early and late dialysate leaks, and incisional hernias.

The subcutaneous section allows a degree of freedom in siting the exit site at a convenient place on the abdominal wall. Simple catheters without cuffs create peritoneal fistulae and predispose to fluid leaks and peritonitis. Such catheters were abandoned after the introduction of

Tenckhoff catheters in 1968, which consist of a body or tubing and two Dacron® cuffs which allow ingrowth of fibrous tissue producing an antibacterial seal. The part of the tube between the two cuffs (5cm long) lies within the tunnel proper, which consists of tissue ingrown into the cuffs and a fibrous sheath covering the intercuff segment of the tube.

The subcutaneous segment is implanted in a way to direct the catheter exit caudally or laterally, which reduces exit-site infection. Implantation of a straight catheter in this manner may increase catheter tip migration or external cuff extrusion as the catheter tends to straighten because of its resilience or shape memory; however, good results with straight catheters are achieved. To obviate this problem, the Swan neck catheter with a 170° bend between the cuffs was devised; however, there is no proven superiority of this catheter over the straight catheter.

Intraperitoneal

This portion should lie in the sump of the pelvis. It is in this part of the catheter that designs vary most and include the following (Figure 2):

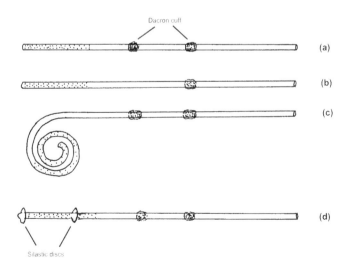

Figure 2 Designs of peritoneal dialysis catheters: a) straight double-cuff Tenckhoff; b) straight single-cuff Tenckhoff; c) curled double-cuff Tenckhoff; d) Oreopoulos-Zellerman (Toronto Western Hospital) catheter.

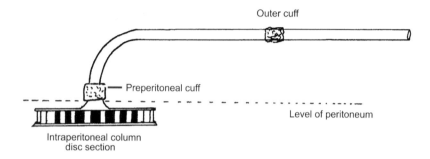

Figure 3 The column disc (Lifecath) catheter.

- straight Tenckhoff with 1mm diameter side holes over the innermost 10cm;
- curled Tenckhoff; a short straight section leading to a curled portion with side holes;
- Oreopoulos-Zellerman (Toronto Western Hospital) which is similar to the straight Tenckhoff but with two intraperitoneal perpendicular discs designed to hold the visceral peritoneum and omentum away from the side holes;
- column disc catheter (Lifecath); two 7cm discs are separated by perpendicular columns which create thin slots through which peritoneal fluid is directed along the parietal peritoneal surface. (Figure 3).

Pre-implantation preparation

The patient should be fully assessed prior to insertion of the CAPD catheter. There are few surgical contraindications for CAPD [2] and these are shown in Table 1. The procedure, including the incidence and nature of complications, should be described to the patient and all questions answered in a reassuring way, allowing a change to haemodialysis if not satisfactory. Prior to insertion, the exit site should be identified and

Table 1 Surgical contraindications to CAPD.

Absolute contraindications

- Extensive intra-abdominal adhesions that limit dialysate flow

- Sepsis of the anterior abdominal wall

- Encapsulating peritoneal sclerosis

- Surgically uncorrectable mechanical defects (e.g. surgically irreparable hernia, omphalocele, gastroschisis, diaphragmatic hernia, and bladder exstrophy)

Relative contraindications

- Fresh intra-abdominal foreign bodies (e.g. 4-month wait after abdominal vascular prostheses, recent ventricular-peritoneal shunt)

- Peritoneal leaks

- Inflammatory, ischaemic bowel disease or frequent episodes of diverticulitis

- Large polycystic kidneys

- Stomas e.g. ileostomy, colostomy

---

marked, which should lie either above or below the belt line, should not lie on a scar, should not be in abdominal folds and should be determined with the patient in an upright position. Bowel preparation with laxatives and the avoidance of constipation are of paramount importance. Similarly, emptying the bladder before the procedure is mandatory. Administration of prophylactic antibiotics (cefuroxime / vancomycin) prevents subsequent catheter infection, peritonitis and wound sepsis.

Placement techniques for CAPD catheters

Catheters must be implanted under strict aseptic technique by a competent and experienced operator in a planned manner, as the attention to detail is paramount for a successful outcome. The area of insertion should be shaved immediately prior to implantation, and the abdominal wall cleaned with povidone-iodine solution and dressed with sterile towels. Immediately before implantation the catheter is removed from the sterile pack and immersed in sterile saline. The Dacron® cuff is wet thoroughly and air squeezed out which provides markedly better tissue ingrowth compared to unwetted, air-containing cuffs. Catheters may be implanted by one of three techniques [3]:

◆ open (surgical);
◆ blind (closed using a Tenckhoff trocar or the Seldindger technique);
◆ peritoneoscopic and laparoscopic insertion.

Open (surgical)

This is the most common method of placement of PD catheters, which is carried out under general, spinal or local anaesthetic, depending upon the fitness of the patient. General anaesthesia is advisable if the patient is obese or has had previous abdominal surgery.

A 5cm vertical incision is made below the umbilicus in the mid-line and deepened through the subcutaneous fat to the linea alba. The linea alba is then divided and extra-peritoneal fat exposed. The peritoneum is then elevated between haemostats and incised at the lowermost end of the incision, and the peritoneal cavity is entered. The catheter is then inserted into the pelvis, either with a pair of sponge-holding forceps or using an introducer, as in the blind or closed technique. The author's preference is for a double-cuff straight Tenckhoff catheter, which is placed by using an in-house purpose-built metallic introducer, as shown in Figure 4. A purse string absorbable suture, including bites of the pre-peritoneal cuff, is used to close the peritoneum, the pre-peritoneal cuff being positioned at the caudal end of the wound just outside the peritoneum. The linea alba is closed over the catheter with continuous absorbable sutures (O PDS), so that it buries 2-3cm of the catheter under the linea alba and snugly encloses the catheter as it passes through it without causing a kink. Proper placement and patency of the catheter is verified by injecting 60ml of saline and observing if 30-40ml is easily aspirated.

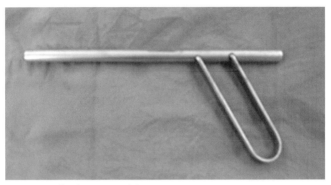

Figure 4 Catheter positioner.

The catheter is tunnelled subcutaneously using a trocar, such that the catheter exits in a caudal direction preventing sweat, water, and dirt flowing down into the exit site. Dissecting the tunnel with artery forceps is traumatic which leads to haematoma formation and infection. The exit-site incision should fit snugly around the catheter. No suture should be placed around the exit site. The skin is closed with an absorbable subcuticular suture. The subcutaneous cuff should be positioned at least 2cm or more from the exit site. The stages of the operation are shown in Figure 5.

Blind (closed: Tenckhoff trocar or Seldinger technique)

The catheter can be inserted either by using a special Tenckhoff trocar or the Seldinger technique. In the former technique, the catheter is inserted through the linea alba under local anaesthesia. It is an inappropriate technique to use where there has been previous lower abdominal surgery or if an ileus is present. A 2-3cm vertical mid-line incision is made below the umbilicus and deepened down to the linea alba. The abdomen is then filled with 500-2000ml of dialysis fluid using a small intravenous cannula. Care is required during this procedure to ensure that the cannula actually enters the peritoneal cavity. Introduction of fluid should be pain-free and if pain or discomfort is experienced at this stage it suggests that fluid may be passing into the pre-peritoneal space.

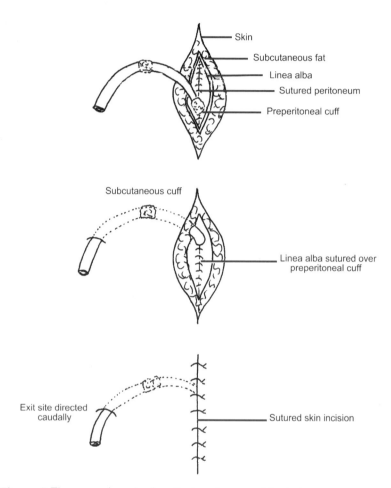

Figure 5 The open (surgical) catheter placement technique.

When fluid priming is complete, the cannula is withdrawn and the assembled Tenckhoff's trocar and cylinder is inserted into the peritoneal cavity through the same hole in the linea alba. To facilitate this, the patient is asked to tense the abdominal muscles. After the peritoneum has been entered, further movement of the trocar will be arrested as its step impinges on the linea alba. On removal of the central part of the trocar, fluid should drain from the tube. The absence of fluid indicates either a pre-peritoneal position or occlusion of the tip of the tube by bowel or omentum. When fluid is seen to drain from the tube, a straight Tenckhoff catheter is mounted on an introducer and is advanced into the trocar tube which is tilted caudally so that the catheter is directed towards the pelvis. The catheter is advanced into the tube until the cuff stops at the narrow portion of the cylinder. The catheter should be seen to drain freely and then the introducer, trocar tube and half cylinders are removed leaving the inner cuff at the level of the linea alba. The subcutaneous tunnel is created exactly as in the open technique.

The closed placement using the Seldinger technique is somewhat similar to the split-sheath technique used for subclavian or internal jugular catheters, which involves passing a guide needle, attached to a syringe with 2-3ml of saline, through the linea alba or the dissected rectus muscle sheath into the peritoneal cavity. The saline is injected into the peritoneal cavity once the 'give' is appreciated, indicating entry into the peritoneal cavity. A Seldinger guidewire is passed through the needle, which is then removed. A tapered dilator with surrounding sheath is passed caudally over the wire, and the dilator is in turn removed. The Tenckhoff catheter is then inserted over the guidewire and the peel-away sheath is split which allows the cuff to advance to a position next to surface of the fascia. With the catheter held in place, the guidewire and the sheath are removed. The catheter is tunnelled subcutaneously as in the open technique.

Peritoneoscopic and laparoscopic insertion

The use of peritoneoscopy for peritoneal catheter placement is a well established technique, where the catheter is inserted under direct vision using a peritoneoscope (Y-Tec) through a single puncture in the mid-line of the abdominal wall. As in the closed technique, a cannula with its trocar is inserted into the peritoneal cavity. The trocar is removed and the peritoneoscope is inserted through the cannula and clear space in the pelvis is identified where the catheter is going to be placed. The remainder of the steps are similar to the Seldinger technique.

Laparoscopic insertion of a PD catheter is usually performed under general anaesthesia. A CO_2 pneumoperitoneum is established and usually two ports are placed for the insertion of the laparoscope and instrumentation. Under vision, the tip of the catheter is advanced through the abdominal cavity into the pelvis and the proximal end of the catheter is then tunnelled subcutaneously to an exit site in the abdomen. Laparoscopy is also utilised to rescue malfunctioning catheters through repositioning, omentectomy and omentopexy [4].

The efficacy and safety of laparoscopic and open insertion of PD catheters have been studied in both randomised and non-randomised studies and there is no significant difference in the overall outcome. The NICE guidance for the routine use of laparoscopic insertion of PD catheter is in the consultation phase.

Complications of catheter insertion

Early complications of catheter insertion

These include [5]:

◆ haemorrhage;
◆ perforated viscus;
◆ wound infection;
◆ catheter obstruction and displacement;
◆ dialysate leakage.

Haemorrhage

This may arise from trauma to the omental or mesenteric vessels, particularly during closed or blind insertion. It may also arise due to extraperitoneal bleeding.

Intraperitoneal bleeding

This usually presents with blood staining of the effluent, which may be heavy. Slight bleeding may be treated expectantly. Heavy bleeding, particularly in association with hypotension, will require a return to theatre for correction.

Extraperitoneal bleeding

This may be obvious with bleeding from the wound edge or an enlarging wound haematoma. Skin edge bleeding can be dealt with by additional sutures. A large wound haematoma should be explored and the source of the bleeding arrested. Failure to evacuate the haematoma predisposes to delayed healing and infection.

Perforated viscus

This is a well recognised hazard of the closed insertion. Rarely does it occur with open insertion. The commonest injuries are bowel and bladder perforation. Evidence of peritonitis associated with contaminated effluent is an indication for laparotomy and repair of the perforation.

Wound infection

Although rare, this is a serious complication, which may jeopardise the success of the catheter. Usual organisms are *Staphylococcus aureus* and Pseudomonas species. Contamination can be prevented by strict adherence to aseptic technique, meticulous haemostasis and prophylactic antibiotics. Treatment of established wound infection requires antibiotics, surgical drainage, and possibly catheter removal.

Catheter obstruction and displacement

Obstruction is one of the commonest problems to affect peritoneal catheters. It usually occurs in the early postoperative period and presents as 'one-way' obstruction (outflow obstruction). Dialysis fluid runs into the peritoneal cavity but drains out slowly or not at all. The commonest cause is usually due to catheter migration from the pelvis to the upper quadrant (Figure 6). Other causes and the management of one-way obstruction are shown in Table 2.

Dialysate leakage

This may occur in up to 25% of catheters placed through the mid-line, but is less with a paramedian or pararectal (Battle) incision. Clinically, leakage presents as a discharge of clear dialysis fluid around the catheter at its exit site or as a localised swelling and oedema of the abdominal wall,

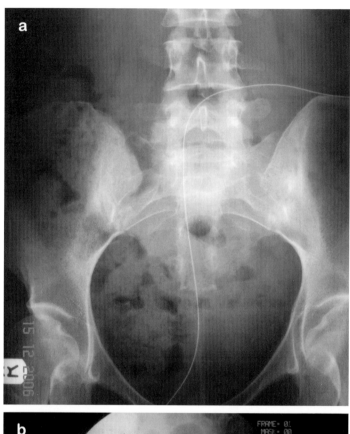

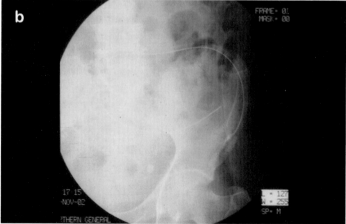

Figure 6 Abdominal X-rays showing: a) normal and b) displaced PD catheters.

Table 2 Causes of management of catheter obstruction.

Cause	Prevention/treatment
Constipation	Relief of constipation
Clot	Syringe flushing Manual pressure to dialysis bag Heparin Thrombolysis, e.g. urokinase
Omental wrap	Omentectomy
Adhesions	Adhesiolysis

Catheter tip migration	Repositioning
	    Fogarty catheter
	    Trocar
	    Laparoscopy
	
	Catheter replacment

which is secondary to infiltration of the abdominal wall with fluid. Genital oedema may also occur. Early leakage can be managed by temporary discontinuation of CAPD. Occasionally catheter replacement is required.

Late complications of catheter insertion

These include:

- exit-site and tunnel infections;
- subcutaneous cuff extrusion;
- catheter obstruction;
- peri-catheter leak;
- peri-catheter hernia;
- encapsulated peritoneal sclerosis (EPS).

Exit-site and tunnel infections

The exit-site infection is defined as the presence of purulent discharge with or without erythema of the skin at the catheter/epidermal interface. Formations of crust around the exit or positive culture in the absence of inflammation do not indicate infection. A tunnel infection may present with erythema, oedema or tenderness over the subcutaneous pathway and usually occurs in combination with exit-site infection. Causes include poor exit-site care and excessive catheter movement, due to traction on the extraperitoneal section of the tube. The most serious and common exit-site pathogens are *Staphylococcus aureus* and *Pseudomonas aeruginosa*, which can lead to peritonitis, hence the need for aggressive treatment with antibiotics until the exit site appears entirely normal. Ultrasonography of the tunnel is essential to evaluate the response to therapy. Exit-site infections progressing to peritonitis or exit-site infection in conjunction with peritonitis are indications for removal of the catheter.

Subcutaneous cuff extrusion

Location of the subcutaneous cuff close to the exit predisposes to its extrusion, which is favoured by the resilience force or the shape memory, and pulling and tugging of the catheter. If the subcutaneous cuff of the peritoneal catheter begins to extrude from the exit site, it may result in persistent exit-site infection. If there are no signs of tunnel or deep (pre-peritoneal) cuff infection, removing the subcutaneous cuff allows the exit infection to resolve in half the cases unresponsive to other treatment. To remove the cuff, first swab the exit site with povidone-iodine solution and then pull on the catheter to expose the cuff through the exit site. Rinse the head of a disposable safety razor in 70% alcohol solution and apply the razor blade to the surface of the cuff, while maintaining tension on the tube, pulling the blade in a direction parallel to the catheter. Rinse the razor head in the 70% alcohol solution to cleanse it and remove all of the cuff until the underlying surface of the catheter is smooth and free from Dacron. Release the catheter allowing it back into the tunnel and swab the exit site with povidone-iodine. If the infection fails to settle, catheter removal is required.

Catheter obstruction

Late catheter obstruction is rare. It may be due to plugging of the tube by omentum, but this tends to be an early rather than a late event. Occasionally in the female, the tube may be blocked by wrapping with the Fallopian tube.

Peri-catheter leak

Dialysis solution leaks may occur months or even years after starting CAPD. Management of a late leak is similar to the one described for an early leak. However, most cases of late leak are refractory to conservative therapy and require surgical treatment. Removal of the tube will be required followed by reinsertion after the old incision has healed.

Peri-catheter hernias

Peri-catheter hernias are difficult to manage without removing the dialysis catheter. Any attempt to repair a peri-catheter hernia leaving the catheter intact will either compromise the hernia repair or the catheter function. Meticulous attention to technique in placement of the catheter will usually prevent hernias developing.

Encapsulated peritoneal sclerosis (EPS)

Encapsulated peritoneal sclerosis (EPS), also termed sclerosing peritonitis, is an unpredictable and devastating complication of PD characterised by fibrosis of the visceral peritoneum, often associated with ascites and extensive intestinal encasement (Figures 6 and 7). In addition to ultrafiltration failure, the patients present with symptoms of persistent, intermittent, or recurrent intestinal obstruction, sometimes associated with bloody effluent or ascites in a patient no longer on PD therapy. Mortality is high and treatment options are inadequate because of poor understanding of the pathogenesis. Whilst there are reports of successful treatment by steroids and total parenteral nutrition therapy, laparotomy is usually required for the relief of intestinal obstruction. Closure of the abdomen may not be possible following laparotomy and a polypropylene mesh may be required. Subsequent PD is inadvisable and rarely possible [6].

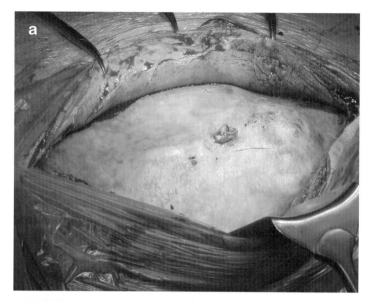

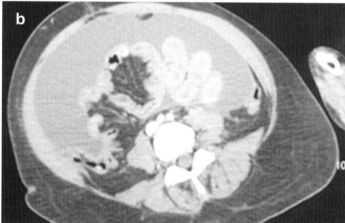

Figure 7 a) Encapsulated peritoneal sclerosis (EPS) at laparotomy showing the thick white membrane beneath the peritoneum. The Tenckhoff catheter passed through the nodule is seen in the centre of the membrane. b) Computerised scan showing EPS.

Surgical problems complicating CAPD

Abdominal wall hernias

It has been estimated that between 10-25% of the CAPD population have hernias. The most common are inguinal, para-umbilical, and peri-catheter hernias. Elective repair should be considered for all other forms of hernia. This may be undertaken without disruption of dialysis if the repair is not extensive, and small volume, short dwell cycles are carried out. If the hernia is large, the patient can be changed to haemodialysis while healing occurs.

Patent processus vaginalis

The passage of dialysis fluid through a patent processus vaginalis may lead to gross scrotal and penile oedema in the male and labial oedema in the female. Sometimes the oedema is so marked that it is not possible to decide from which side the leak is coming. The performance of an isotope peritoneo-scrotogram using technetium will delineate the side of the lesion. Prior to repair of the patent processus vaginalis, CAPD should be discontinued until the oedema has subsided and then the processus vaginalis should be located and closed. The patient should be converted to haemodialysis and then CAPD may be instituted about two weeks following repair.

Organ erosion

A catheter in the abdomen without dialysate can cause organ erosion, particularly bowel, vagina and bladder, hence the importance of early removal of unused catheters [7].

Surgical aspects of peritonitis

In some cases the surgical assessment of the CAPD patient who has an acute abdomen is difficult [8]. The question must be asked in that is the aetiology of the peritonitis related to the CAPD? i.e. CAPD peritonitis or is it related to a problem arising with inflammation or perforation of an intra-abdominal organ? Acute abdominal emergencies, e.g. cholecystitis and appendicitis may occasionally be difficult to diagnose in patients on CAPD and it may be extremely difficult to distinguish them from CAPD peritonitis. Poor response of presumed CAPD peritonitis to antibiotics, or the isolation of multiple organisms, especially Gram-negative organisms and anaerobes, may indicate a primary abdominal pathology rather than CAPD peritonitis. However, the presence of particulate matter, bile or faeces in the CAPD effluent will make the diagnosis of a perforated viscus obvious. A high amylase in CAPD fluid will suggest a diagnosis of acute pancreatitis.

If emergency surgery is required and there is gross bacterial contamination of the peritoneal cavity, e.g. faecal peritonitis, the CAPD tube should be removed and the patient commenced on haemodialysis postoperatively, the CAPD tube being reinserted at a later date when sepsis has abated and the abdominal wall healed. However, with perforated peptic ulceration where the peritonitis is of a chemical nature, the CAPD tube may be left *in situ*, haemodialysis being instituted until healing has occurred when CAPD may be re-established.

CAPD peritonitis refractory to antibiotic treatment for five days and those caused by Pseudomonas, Candida and Mycobacterium should be treated with removal of the catheter to protect the peritoneal membrane for future use [9].

Routine non-emergency surgery in CAPD patients

The practice varies for patients on CAPD who are undergoing abdominal surgery. One of the following practices may be adopted:

◆   removal of the Tenckhoff catheter at the time of surgery with institution of haemodialysis via a double-lumen internal jugular catheter until abdominal healing has occurred (3-6 weeks), with subsequent reinsertion of the Tenckhoff catheter. Following this regime, difficulty may be encountered at the time of reinserting the catheter due to adhesions;

◆ retention of the Tenckhoff catheter but with institution of haemodialysis until abdominal wall healing has occurred (3-6 weeks), with resumption of CAPD with the Tenckhoff catheter. Infection of the Tenckhoff catheter may occur with this method and the catheter may need to be removed;

◆ retention of the Tenckhoff catheter using small exchanges of dialysis fluid on a 'cycling' machine (continuous cycling peritoneal dialysis), until the abdominal wall is healed (10-12 weeks), when full two-litre volume exchanges are resumed. This method is only applicable if a contaminated viscus is not breached, e.g. hernia repair or division of adhesions.

For routine non-emergency surgery, e.g. cholecystectomy, colectomy (without stoma formation), the authors' preference is for retention of the CAPD tube using covering antibiotics and utilising haemodialysis for 2-3 weeks and then re-instituting CAPD via the in-dwelling Tenckhoff catheter.

Indications for catheter removal

The indications for catheter removal are shown in Table 3. The authors' preference is to remove the catheter under local anaesthetic unless the patient is obese or there is abdominal wall sepsis or oedema. If the patient is not already on antibiotics, prophylactic antibiotics are administered. The catheter is approached by re-opening the old primary incision over the deep cuff. Careful attention to haemostasis is essential. Using sharp dissection the Dacron cuffs are freed from the surrounding tissue. It is important to remove all portions of the Dacron cuffs. Residual Dacron may serve as a nidus for chronic infection. Great care must be exercised while removing the pre-peritoneal cuff to avoid injury to the bowel. Peritoneal and linea alba defects are closed with absorbable sutures. The skin is closed with a subcuticular absorbable suture, unless the wound is grossly infected when it is left open and packed.

Catheter replacement

The commonest causes for catheter removal are an infected exit site, tunnel infection, and peritonitis not responding to adequate treatment. For

Table 3 Indications for catheter removal.

Malfunction

- Obstruction with blood clot, fibrin or omental incarceration

- Catheter tip migration with poor drainage

- Catheter kinking

- Catheter tip caught in adhesions following peritonitis

- Catheter breakage

Functioning catheter with complications

- Recurrent attacks of CAPD peritonitis

- Persistent exit-site infection

- Tunnel infection/abscess

- Loss of ultrafiltration

- Late leaks

- Bowel perforation with multiple organism peritonitis

- Unusual forms of peritonitis, e.g. fungal, TB, sclerosing

Functioning catheter no longer needed

- Transfer to haemodialysis

- Post-renal transplantation

---

exit-site and tunnel infection, catheter replacement can be carried out 1-2 weeks after catheter removal, usually through a different site. If the catheter has to be removed for frequent recurrence of peritonitis with the same organism or other infected causes, then the catheter can usually be reinserted after three weeks of termination of successful treatment of the peritonitis. Replacement of catheters at the same time as removal has been reported [10] . The authors have used this method successfully, but it is probably unwise to use it in patients with fungal, mycobacterial or faecal infections. When replacing a catheter it is appropriate to use a different site.

Transplantation in patients on CAPD

A patient on CAPD undergoing renal transplantation may face an extra risk of infection from the peritoneal cavity and the catheter. It is the authors' practice to avoid transplantation if the patient has active CAPD peritonitis. Exit-site infection does not preclude transplantation but it may be appropriate to remove the catheter at the time of the transplant with careful isolation of the two wounds to avoid cross infection. The patient would require to be converted to haemodialysis if delayed function of the transplant occurred.

Preparation for transplantation

Patients presenting for cadaveric transplantation must be prepared for theatre in a very short time, usually under 12 hours. If the patient is on CAPD, the date of previous episodes of peritonitis and exit-site infection need to be known, as do any difficulties with drainage or poor dialysis. A sample of CAPD fluid should be centrifuged and examined for white cells or organisms using a Gram stain. Fluid should also be sent for culture. Prior to surgery, the peritoneum should be emptied of CAPD fluid.

Intra-operative management

The catheter and exit sites should be excluded from the operation site by surgical drapes. In a patient undergoing a first transplant, it is usually appropriate to use the opposite iliac fossa to that of the exit site. Care must be taken to avoid breaching the peritoneum when exposing the iliac vessels. If a small hole is made in the peritoneum, it should be repaired in a watertight fashion. After the transplant wound has been closed and dressed, the CAPD tube may be removed if there is any specific indication for removal. The authors remove the catheters routinely following live donor renal transplantation, as the transplant is expected to function immediately.

Postoperative management

The catheter should be left *in situ* for 2-3 months post-transplant, as it may be temporarily required for dialysis if function of the transplanted kidney is delayed. Also, if the graft is going to be lost due to acute rejection the majority are usually lost within the first 2-3 months post-transplant. Catheter care during this period must be meticulous. Regular cultures of CAPD fluid should be taken during this period if CAPD is required post-transplant. If episodes of CAPD peritonitis occur, they should be treated conventionally but there should be a low threshold for removal of the catheter and conversion to haemodialysis. Once graft function is established, the CAPD tube should be clamped and capped. The catheter should be removed electively after 2-3 months when graft function is stable.

Conclusions

As peritoneal catheters are lifelines for PD patients, meticulous surgical technique with attention to detail and post-implantation care are paramount in achieving trouble-free and long-term access to the peritoneal cavity. A dedicated and experienced team consisting of nephrologists, surgeons and nurses is required for satisfactory management of peritoneal access. The complications related to PD catheters should be recognised early and treated promptly, maintaining a low threshold for their removal. The results and complications of surgery should be reported and audited in the standard fashion.

Key Summary

◆ Severe adhesions, encapsulated peritoneal sclerosis, abdominal wall sepsis, inflammatory bowel disease and irreparable hernias absolutely contraindicate CAPD.

◆ There is no evidence to suggest superiority of one catheter over another. However, the double-cuff Tenckhoff catheter is the most widely used catheter.

◆ Placement can be by surgical, percutaneous or laparoscopic techniques so that the tip of the intra-peritoneal part of the catheter should be in the pelvis.

◆ Early complications include haemorrhage, perforated viscus, infection, catheter displacement or obstruction and dialysate leakage.

◆ CAPD peritonitis and acute abdominal emergencies may be differentiated by the bacteriological and biochemical examination of the dialysate.

◆ Infection may require catheter removal if it fails to settle with antibiotics.

◆ Catheter obstruction or persistent peri-catheter leakage require replacement of the tube.

◆ Abdominal wall hernias require urgent repair.

◆ Catheter survival of >80% at one year is a reasonable goal.

References

1. Twardiwski ZJ. Peritoneal dialysis glossary. II. *Perit Dial Int* 1988; 8: 15-7.
2. Shetty A, Oreopoulos DG. Peritoneal dialysis: its indications and contraindications. *Dialysis and Transplantation* 2000; 29(2): 71-7.
3. Twardowski ZJ, Nichols WK. Peritoneal dialysis access and exit-site care including surgical aspects. *Text Book of Peritoneal dialysis.* Gokal R, Khanna R, *et al*, Eds. London: Kluwer Academic Publication, 2000: Chapter 9.
4. Wright MJ, Bel'eed K, Johnson BF, *et al*. Randomised prospective comparison of laparoscopic and open peritoneal dialysis catheter insertion. *Perit Dial Int* 1999; 19(4): 372-5.
5. Gokal R, Alexander S, Ash S, *et al*. Peritoneal catheters and exit-site practices toward optimum peritoneal access: 1998 update. (Official report from the International Society for Peritoneal Dialysis). *Perit Dial Int* 1998; 18(1): 11-33.
6. Chin AI, Yeun JY. Encapsulating peritoneal sclerosis: an unpredictable and devastating complication of peritoneal dialysis. *Am J Kidney Dis* 2006; 47(4): 697-712.
7. Shrestha BM, Wilkie M, Raftery AT. Delayed perforation of colon caused by an unused peritoneal dialysis catheter presenting with diarrhoea. *Perit Dial Int* 2003; 23 (6): 610-1.
8. Miller GV, Bhandari S, Brownjohn AM, *et al*. 'Surgical' peritonitis in the CAPD patient. *Ann R Coll Surg Eng* 1998; 80: 36-9.
9. Piraino B, Bailie GR, Bernardini J, *et al*. ISPD guidelines/recommendations on peritoneal dialysis-related infections; recommendations: 2005 update. *Perit Dial Int* 2005; 25: 107-31.
10. Paterson AD, Bishop MC, Morgan AG, *et al*. Removal and replacement of Tenckhoff catheter at a single operation: successful treatment of resistant peritonitis in continuous ambulatory peritoneal dialysis. *Lancet* 1986; 2: 1245-7.

Chapter 16

Vascular access in children

Pierre Bourquelot MD

Vascular Access Surgeon, Vascular Access Department, Clinique Jouvenet, Paris, France

Microsurgery gives much better immediate and long-term results than classical surgery for the creation of direct arteriovenous fistulae, the best chronic access to blood in children [1].

Introduction

First described by Brescia and Cimino in 1966, the autogenous arteriovenous (AV) fistula was soon considered as the best form of haemodialysis angio-access in adults. In children the first publications indicated 50% immediate failure due to small vessels, often reduced by spasm provoked by arterial dissection. In 1960, Jacobson and Suarez achieved the first vascular micro-anastomosis on 1mm-diameter vessels. When applied to AV fistula creation in children, microsurgery provides a dramatic benefit. Other forms of angio-access may have deleterious effects on children: central venous catheters (CVC) may cause central vein stenosis and thrombosis, precluding further AV fistula formation, and arteriovenous grafts (AVG) have very poor patency in children. Finally, renal transplantation may not last a lifetime. For children with access created for diseases other than end-stage renal disease (ESRD), the microsurgical creation of an AV fistula is also a safe and durable alternative to peripheral venipuncture and CVC.

Microsurgical technique

Preservation of the veins is essential in every child requiring haemodialysis. Whenever possible, the dorsal veins of the hand must be used for blood sampling. Absolute protection of the non-dominant arm is necessary. Subclavian CVCs, which have a high risk of proximal upper limb venous stenosis, should be prohibited. The condition of the vein is assessed by careful pre-operative clinical examination: a duplex scan is necessary if there is any doubt, particularly in very young children; and venous angiography is mandatory in patients who have previously had a CVC. A prophylactic broad spectrum antibiotic is prescribed. The rules for suturing are that forceps must never grasp the intima, the adventitia is incised and not resected, high pressure clamps must be avoided, and the thinnest possible needles are to be used. Preventive haemostasis using a pneumatic tourniquet [2] makes extensive arterial dissection for clamping unnecessary: arterial spasm is avoided. When haemostasis is incomplete,

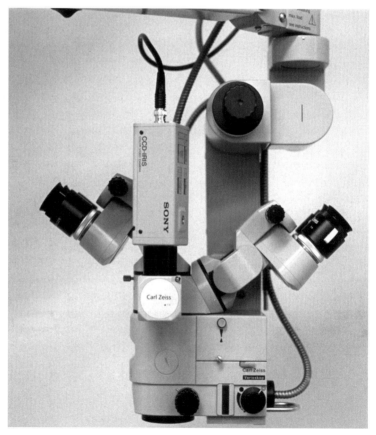

Figure 1 Surgical microscope.

microclamps are placed on the artery after minimal dissection. Anticoagulation is mandatory in hypercoagulation conditions (mainly nephrotic syndrome). The equipment needed includes: ophthalmologic scissors, microsurgical needle holders, a disposable ophthalmologic scalpel, Dumont forceps, single and double Acland clamps, heparinised saline, a surgical microscope (Figure 1) with two facing binoculars, and Ethilon 9-10/0 (BV70 - BV50) sutures.

Radiocephalic arteriovenous fistulae (Figures 2 and 3)

The incision is longitudinal, half way between the cephalic vein and the radial artery in the wrist. The nerves must be carefully preserved. The vein is freed, a ligature being placed on the collateral branches avoiding electric coagulation that could damage the vascular trunk itself. Saline irrigation must be frequent in order to prevent drying, and vessels are only handled by the adventitia. After section of the vein above a ligature, a longitudinal posterior incision of approximately 10mm in length is made in the proximal vein. The anterior wall of the artery is exposed. A longitudinal arteriotomy is made with a disposable ophthalmologic scalpel and

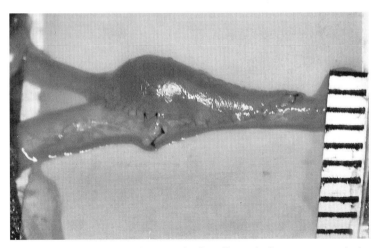

Figure 2 Completed microsurgical radiocephalic anastomosis in an infant.

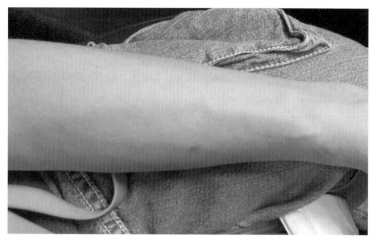

Figure 3 Functioning radiocephalic AV fistula in a 13-year-old child, one month postoperatively.

completed with scissors. If a few drops of blood appear they are rinsed with heparin saline and dried with small sponges. The anastomosis is constructed with four continuous sutures, starting with the proximal angle. The continuous suture is left loose at the beginning so as to leave the lumen open. Frequent use of the zoom facilitates this very precise part of the operation and the needle must be repositioned in the needle holder for each passage through a vessel. The two proximal continuous sutures (posterior and anterior) are inserted as far as the middle of the arteriotomy. The anastomosis is completed starting from the distal angle. The tourniquet is then released. If there is a leak, an additional suture is added. Patency is confirmed by Doppler ultrasound, as the murmur can be absent during the first postoperative hours, particularly in small children. It is very important to ascertain that the vein is not stenosed at the upper limit of the dissection.

Variations

A variation in technique is to use a single running suture for the anastomosis. The proximal suture is performed first, starting at the middle of the posterior wall of the arteriotomy, proceeding to the proximal angle, and down to the middle of the anterior wall. The distal suture is then completed. This technique gives excellent vision of the arterial lumen. It may be necessary to surgically transpose the vein subcutaneously two months later in small children with thick subcutaneous tissue.

Ulnobasilic arteriovenous fistulae

A sufficient length of the vein must be freed, as it is situated at a distance from the artery. It can be helpful to place the forearm in flexion at the elbow during dissection. The artery is approached by partial excision of the flexor carpi ulnaris. A longer maturation period is required before needling than for radiocephalic AV fistulae.

Brachiocephalic arteriovenous fistulae

A transverse incision at the anterior aspect of the elbow exposes the medial branch of the cephalic vein, which must be sufficiently freed to allow it to come into proximity with the brachial artery without traction. Here again, using a pneumatic tourniquet avoids having to free the artery.

Variations

An anastomosis between the brachial artery and the cephalic vein via the medial branch of the basilic vein is preferable. This will be perfused backwards in the absence of valves. Both vessels, which follow almost superimposed routes, are approached by a short antecubital incision. The vein is divided as high as possible and, after minimal dissection, its lower segment is anastomosed to the brachial artery. It is essential to ligate the perforating antecubital vein to avoid the risk of high flow with cardiac overload. Ligation of the distal cephalic vein in the upper forearm is also necessary to avoid the risk of retrograde perfusion of the forearm, which would impair venous drainage of the hand. For similar reasons retrograde AV fistulae and side-to-side AV fistulae at the elbow should be avoided.

Brachiobasilic arteriovenous fistulae with subcutaneous transposition

The basilic vein follows a route which rapidly becomes deep above the elbow, so that it is often undamaged. Its use for angio-access necessitates surgical transposition, even in the thinnest children. Its transposition is much easier when it is performed during a second stage, the first consisting of a simple AV fistula at the elbow which results in dilatation of the vein and thickening of its walls. The initial AV fistula is constructed using the medial branch of the basilic vein at the elbow or, if necessary, its lateral branch. Transposition performed two months later requires a longitudinal incision on the medial side of the upper arm. Collaterals of the veins are ligated and divided. The vein is tunnelled very superficially along a straight line. Reimplantation on the artery is performed as low as possible. An interval of three weeks must be left before puncturing.

Femorofemoral arteriovenous fistulae, with transposition

This type of vascular access is rarely used. Superficial transposition of the femoral vein is usually in a straight line with an anastomosis on the distal superficial femoral artery.

Arteriovenous bridge grafts

In this case a graft (biograft or PTFE) is implanted between an artery and a vein. It is located under the skin in such a way as to be accessible to puncture.

The results of microsurgical AV fistula creation

Without microsurgery

Limited-quality AV fistulae are frequently observed (Table 1). Proximal fistulae and grafts are easier to construct in children but they have high complication rates, will destroy proximal veins and, therefore, threaten the

Table 1 Arteriovenous angio-access in children: major publications.

	Bourquelot[7]	Sanabia	Lumsden	Bagolan	Sheth[4]	Ramage[5]
Year of publication	1990	1993	1994	1998	2002	2005
Country	France	Spain	USA	Italy	USA	UK
Microsurgery	yes	yes	no	yes	no	no
Number of accesses	434	86	61	112	52	107
Failing to mature AV fistula	10%	10%	30%	5%	33%	-
AV fistula vs. graft	93%	100%	24%	100%	46%	84%

long-term survival of the patient. In 1994, Lumdsen reported on 61 angio-accesses in children without microsurgery; the mean age was 11 years, only 25% were simple AV fistulae and 30% of them failed to mature [3]. The mean functional patency was 6.2 months; 76% of the accesses were grafts, mostly in the upper arm or in the thigh, with a mean patency of ten months. In 2002, Sheth [4] reported on 52 arteriovenous angio-accesses in 13-year-old (mean age) children. The percentage of autogenous AV fistulae was low (46%) and the percentage of primary failures (failed to mature) was high (33%).

Curiously, these two authors demonstrated no interest in microsurgery and made no reference to any of the previous publications concerning microsurgical creation of AV fistulae in children. Furthermore, Sheth stated wrongly that "the literature contains very little data regarding the success of permanent vascular access in paediatric patients". In fact, the three European surgical teams who used microsurgery for angio-accesses creation in children (Table 1) reported only 5-10% of fistulae that failed to mature compared to 30-33% observed by the two American teams who were not using microsurgery. Similarly, the percentages of autogenous AV fistulae creation versus grafts decreased from 86-100% with microsurgery to 24-46% without microsurgery.

In 2005, Ramage [5] published the results of a 20-year retrospective study without the use of microsurgery. One hundred and twenty-two arteriovenous vascular access procedures were performed on children, with a median age at initial access formation of 12 years (range, four weeks to 21 years). The most common procedure was CVC insertion (n=182) and then AV fistula formation (n=107), with only 15 AVGs created. Median censored survival was 3.14 years (95% confidence interval, 1.22 to 5.06) for AV fistulae and 0.6 years (95% confidence interval, 0.20 to 1.00) for CVCs. Factors adversely affecting vascular access survival were younger age, trainee operator, presence of hypoalbuminemia, and type of access undertaken, with AV fistulae shown to be better than CVCs.

With microsurgery

Our first experience for AV fistulae in 32 children (Table 1) was reported in 1978 (Coulonges S, Thèse de Médecine, Université Pierre et Marie Curie Paris VI) and we published our first results for AV fistula microsurgery in children under 10kg in 1981 [6]. In 1990 [7], we reported 380 children undergoing microsurgery: 93% were autogenous AV fistulae and only 7% were prosthetic bridge grafts, with 78% of patients having a distal autogenous fistula. The immediate patency rate was 96% and the 24-month patency rate was 85% in distal radiocephalic fistulae, 72% in brachiobasilic fistulae, 47% in brachiocephalic fistulae and only 5% in bridge grafts (Figure 4).

These benefits of microsurgery for children have been emphasised by a Canadian group (Yazbeck) in 1984, by Spanish workers in 1993 (Sanabia) and by an Italian team in 1998 (Bagolan).

In a survey of the three paediatric nephrology departments in Paris on 1 February 2003, we observed that 70% of 33 ESRD children were being haemodialysed via an autogenous fistula, 24% via a jugular CVC, and 6% were on peritoneal dialysis. This compared favourably with the annual publication of the North American Pediatric Renal Transplant Cooperative (NAPRTC) Study in 1996 [8] reporting that between 1 January 1992 and 16 January 1996 two-thirds of children and adolescents on dialysis were

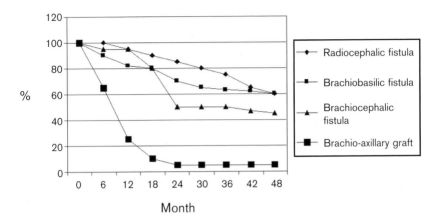

Figure 4 Angio-access in children: long-term patency (n=434).

maintained on peritoneal dialysis, despite an overall peritonitis rate of one episode every 13 patient-months, and the majority of haemodialysis accesses were external percutaneous catheters (Figure 5), with the subclavian vein the most common site. More recently the publication of NAPRTC in 2003 [9] reported that, between 1992 and 1998, 70-80% of

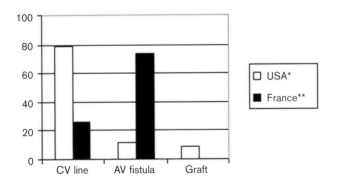

Figure 5 Percentages of central venous catheter vs. arteriovenous access in American and French children. (* 2001 NAPRTCS report; ** Paris 01/02/2003).

children and 59% of adolescents on dialysis were maintained on peritoneal dialysis, and that younger children received haemodialysis, almost exclusively through percutaneous catheters, while 57% of children more than six years old were dialysed with a fistula or graft after six months on haemodialysis.

In 2001, we retrospectively reviewed 69 AV fistulae in a young (mean age 20 years) and difficult cohort of 64 non-renal chronic disease patients requiring a permanent angio-access for repeated transfusions, perfusions, apheresis and drug injections for sickle cell anaemia, parenteral nutrition,

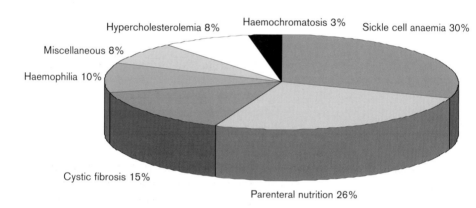

Figure 6 Pathologies of non-ESRD patients undergoing AV fistula formation.

cystic fibrosis, haemophilia, hypercholesterolemia, haemochromatosis, and miscellaneous conditions (Figure 6). Although there had been no previous venous preservation strategy, it was possible with microsurgery to create distal AV fistulae in 68% of cases; insertion of a graft was necessary in only 4%. The long-term patency rate was around 60% after ten years (Figure 7).

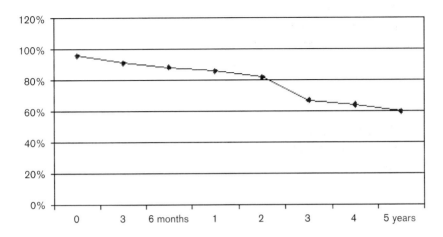

Figure 7 Long-term patency of autogenous arteriovenous fistulae in 64 non-renal chronic disease young patients.

Conclusions

Microsurgery is mandatory for the creation of angio-access in children. It provides a dramatic improvement in the construction of distal versus proximal autogenous AV fistulae, with better immediate and long-term results. Microsurgery will avoid the need for grafts, whose mid-term patency is poor, and central venous catheters, which carry a major risk of central venous stenosis. Children with pathologies other than ESRD that require long-term repeated access to the circulation may also benefit from the creation of AV fistulae.

Key Summary

◆ Microsurgery is a prerequisite for creation of angio-access in children. It includes the use of a surgical microscope, microsurgical instruments, prophylactic haemostasis and no-touch surgery.

◆ In recent publications, the percentages of arteriovenous fistulae versus grafts varied from 34-46% without microsurgery, and from 86-100% with microsurgery. Likewise, the percentages of AV fistulae which failed to mature varied from 30-33% without microsurgery, and from 5-10% with microsurgery.

◆ Good results of microsurgically created AV fistulae partly explain the high percentage of end-stage renal disease (ESRD) children treated by haemodialysis in Paris using an autogenous fistula (70% of 33 children), while only 24% were haemodialysed via a central venous catheter and 6% were on peritoneal dialysis.

◆ Microsurgical AV fistulae are also created successfully in children requiring frequent access to the circulation for various non-ESRD chronic diseases. We were able to create a distal AV fistula in 68% of cases and the long-term patency rate was just below 60% after ten years.

References

1.   Bourquelot P. Vascular access in children: the importance of microsurgery for creation of autologous arteriovenous fistulae. *Eur J Vasc Endovasc Surg* 2006; 32: 696-700.
2.   Bourquelot P. Preventive haemostasis with an inflatable tourniquet for microsurgical distal arteriovenous fistulas for haemodialysis. *Microsurgery* 1993; 14: 462-3.

3. Lumsden AB, Macdonald MJ, Allen RC, Dodson TF. Hemodialysis access in the pediatric patient population. *Am J Surg* 1994; 168: 197-201.

4. Sheth RD, Brandt ML, Brewer ED, *et al.* Permanent hemodialysis vascular access survival in children and adolescents with end-stage renal disease. *Kidney Int* 2002; 62: 1864-9.

5. Ramage IJ, Bailie A, Tyerman KS, *et al.* Vascular access survival in children and young adults receiving long-term hemodialysis. *Am J Kidney Dis* 2005; 45: 708-14.

6. Bourquelot P, Wolfeler L, Lamy L. Microsurgery for haemodialysis distal arteriovenous fistulae in children weighing less than 10kg. *Proc Eur Dial Transplant Assoc* 1981; 18: 537-41.

7. Bourquelot P, Cussenot O, Corbi P, *et al.* Microsurgical creation and follow-up of arteriovenous fistulae for chronic haemodialysis in children. *Pediatr Nephrol* 1990; 4: 156-9.

8. Lerner GR, Warady BA, Sullivan EK, Alexander SR. Chronic dialysis in children and adolescents. The 1996 annual report of the North American Pediatric Renal Transplant Cooperative Study. *Pediatr Nephrol* 1999; 13: 404-17.

9. Leonard MB, Donaldson LA, Ho M, Geary DF. A prospective cohort study of incident maintenance dialysis in children: an NAPRTC study. *Kidney Int* 2003; 63(2): 744-55.

Chapter 17

The role of the vascular access nurse specialist

Alison J Cornall RN BA (Hons) MSc

Vascular Access Nurse Specialist, Churchill Hospital, Oxford, UK

Paula A Davies RN

Vascular Access Nurse Specialist, Morriston Hospital, Swansea, UK

The rationale for the vascular access nurse specialist

Vascular access failure is the most common cause of morbidity and hospitalisation among dialysis patients worldwide, and remains the Achilles heel of patients with end-stage renal disease (ESRD) who are receiving haemodialysis (HD). Adequate delivery of prescribed HD relies on an optimally functioning vascular access. The creation and maintenance of vascular access for HD is becoming more difficult, due to the increasing number of elderly dialysis patients with additional cardiovascular comorbidities and diabetes mellitus [1].

Establishing effective access for HD is therefore a significant responsibility in renal units, already struggling to treat an increasing number of aging dialysis patients. The national trend has been a year on year increase in the HD population and an increase in those using arteriovenous (AV) fistulae. In the UK, this rise is predicted to continue until at least 2020. The UK Renal Registry Report (2005) estimated that over 37,800 adult patients received renal replacement therapy in the UK at the end of 2004 [2].

The provision of dialysis treatment is a challenge in itself, but the provision and maintenance of vascular access adds a substantial associated and unrecognised extra workload for the surgical, radiological and nephrology teams. Additional procedures are needed when patients present with complications, such as thrombosis, infection, stenosis and unsatisfactory access performance [3].

In an attempt to resolve some of the difficulties surrounding the provision of dialysis vascular access, an increasing number of renal units in the UK have employed vascular access nurse specialists (VANS) to improve the service delivery. The aim of such posts is to co-ordinate existing resources to achieve greater efficiency, better continuity and improved quality of patient care. The role is ideally suited to nurses with particular expertise in dialysis, who can liaise easily with surgical, radiological and medical teams. The posts are continuing to evolve and vary in detail, depending on local needs, but in each case the overall aim is to maximise the quantity and quality of natural vascular access with an emphasis on increasing the number of AV fistulae. The success of the VANS role depends on achieving a good rapport and optimal communication with the members of the multidisciplinary team.

Fundamental components of the VANS role include:

◆ co-ordination and planning of the vascular access pathway;
◆ maintenance and surveillance of existing vascular access;
◆ advanced clinical practice procedures;
◆ education; and
◆ clinical audit.

Co-ordination and planning of the vascular access pathway

The benefits of good vascular access are now widely recognised and targets are being set to improve standards. The UK Renal National Service framework (NSF), part one, standard 3 states:

"All children, young people and adults with established renal failure are to have timely and appropriate surgery for permanent vascular or peritoneal dialysis access, which is monitored and maintained to achieve its maximum longevity." [4]

The revised Renal Association guidelines on vascular access identify that "at least 65% of patients presenting more than three months before initiation of dialysis should start HD with a usable native arteriovenous fistula" [5].

The updated DOQI clinical practice guidelines for vascular access recommend that "a fistula should be placed six months before the anticipated start of HD treatments. This timing allows for access evaluation and additional time for revision to ensure a working fistula is available at the initiation of dialysis therapy" [6].

Meeting such targets is not straightforward, but is achievable with better organisation of the entire vascular access pathway. Such a pathway needs to define both sequence and timing of events leading to access placement and should also embody standards against which performance can be audited [3] (Figure 1).

The most important component of the VANS role is management of the referral process. Patient prioritisation can be more equitable and there is the potential for the creation of a single access waiting list. Theatre lists are then co-ordinated, and organised independently and flexibly so that patients may be prioritised on the basis of clinical need. This makes it possible to expedite the surgery of patients who present acutely in ESRD or those whose renal function deteriorates faster than previously anticipated. In the same way, it is possible to accelerate pre-operative investigations and the revision of established access. The time from referral to surgery, the number of clinic visits and the wait for investigations are greatly reduced. Such delays are well recognised contributors to the delay in creating permanent vascular access in the ESRD population in the UK [3].

A level of autonomy allows the VANS to see vascular access referrals on the wards and dialysis units, order radiological investigations and run outpatient clinics. This level of responsibility requires careful training, assessment of competence and close collaboration between key members of the multidisciplinary team.

Maintenance and surveillance of existing vascular access

The second part of the role is the management of a regular surveillance program, which is two-fold, involving the pre-dialysis and the chronic HD

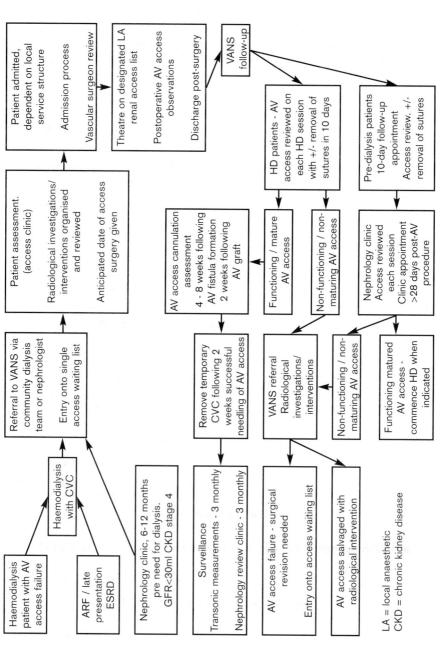

Figure 1 Pathway for vascular access surgery and surveillance.

patient population. AV fistulae vary enormously from patient to patient. Monitoring the development of a newly placed AV fistula by simple inspection, palpation and auscultation should be undertaken on each visit, whether this is a clinic attendance or a routine HD session. A non-functioning/non-maturing AV fistula needs early identification to allow for timely intervention.

If indicated, patients are referred for radiological imaging by the VANS. The initial assessment for AV fistulae and AV grafts is either by duplex ultrasound scanning or fistulography. These techniques permit imaging of vessels to identify stenoses, and have become the gold standard for the initial assessment of fistulae and grafts.

The VANS also co-ordinates and organises plans for intervention by the radiologist or the vascular surgeon. It can be argued that surgical revision remains the best treatment for access stenosis. Alternatively, fistuloplasty, with or without stenting, can postpone the definitive loss of a vascular segment for access use [7]. However, the choice between surgery and interventional radiology is partly dependent on local expertise, resources and anatomical factors.

Falling blood flow rates on HD should initiate intervention. Specific apparatus, such as the Transonic system, is available to measure access flow and recirculation within a regular program of measurements. This is based on the ultrasound dilution technique and the inversion of the inlet and outlet dialyser bloodlines. It is recommended that "investigation of the AV fistula or graft to assess for evidence of arterial or venous stenoses or access recirculation is required if there is a significant fall in the blood flow rate that can be achieved, a reduction in delivered dialysis dose or a persistent rise in venous pressure in sequential dialysis sessions" [5].

The VANS expedites the entire process for those patients whose AV fistulae or AV grafts are at risk of early thrombosis. A consequence of a surveillance program is the identification of a cohort of patients requiring regular venoplasty for central stenoses to maintain their AV fistulae. Over time this conservative strategy reduces the number of long-term haemodialysis patients who have exhausted their sites for natural access.

Advanced clinical practice procedures

Many haemodialysis patients in the UK rely on central venous catheters (CVC) for vascular access, with more than 30% continuing to be dialysed via a CVC [8]. Their use should be strictly monitored and where possible should not replace definitive long-term access provision. Correct insertion of CVCs, their everyday use and follow-up care have an important influence on morbidity and mortality [9]. Consultant nephrologists often provide training, through continuous competency-based assessment. Internal jugular and femoral veins are used for CVC insertion, using real-time two-dimensional ultrasound guidance [5]. Subclavian vein cannulation is associated with central vein stenosis and thrombosis, so this is only considered when all other options are exhausted.

Historically, surgeons, radiologists and nephrologists have provided vascular access for haemodialysis. An innovative part of the VANS role is the insertion of short and long-term CVCs for haemodialysis. It is essential that the VANS has the same education and expertise that would be expected from a doctor employed in the same role; therefore, a comprehensive training program is required. The service provided by the VANS has a positive effect on service delivery. It has the advantage of freeing up the time of medical staff. Efficient access and an uneventful dialysis session with discharge home at the end of the day, reduces patient waiting times and possible hospital admissions [10].

The use of CVCs is inevitable in patients who present late in ESRD or with acute renal failure (ARF). To increase the proportion of patients dialysing with AV fistulae, the VANS is involved in the assessment for both AV fistula formation and early diagnosis of problems that will require either radiological or surgical intervention. This requires specialised knowledge of the anatomy, physiology and pathology of access, together with clinical skills and experience for the diagnosis and appropriate patient referral for intervention. Assessments may take place either in the outpatient department setting or the haemodialysis unit. They involve history taking, physical assessment, making diagnoses, as well as identifying and initiating treatment for infection, poor flows, failing access and post-surgery follow-up.

Education

The VANS role involves the education of patients, family, nurses, and multidisciplinary team members, including theatre and radiology staff.

Patient education begins before vascular access procedures are performed. The importance of vein preservation cannot be emphasised enough, especially in patients at potential risk of developing ESRD. It is well documented that scarring is associated with vein puncture. As a result of this, complications such as stenosis and flow turbulence occur. Ideally, the veins of both arms, not only the dominant arm, should remain untouched. The dorsum of the hand should be favoured for intravenous infusions, and phlebotomy and the cephalic vein must be avoided for drips and venepuncture where possible [6, 11]. Patient booklets and leaflets reinforce information and advice about AV fistula formation and aftercare.

Education continues on the dialysis unit for patients and staff. Frequently, vascular access nurse specialists are responsible for needling complicated or immature AV fistulae because of their extensive knowledge and expertise. Written guidelines and protocols support and reinforce all aspects of vascular access care throughout the renal units to ensure consistency and maintenance of high quality care. Formal education sessions involve lectures and small group teaching.

Clinical audit

Clinical audit influences the planning of service delivery and provides feedback for clinical standards and targets. The audits include a prospective record of the surgical referral pathway in terms of number of referrals and time taken, ultimate performance of the haemodialysis access, and complication rates such as CVC infection rates. A prospective audit of radiological interventions is used to evaluate the results of different methods of radiological intervention, according to vascular access and site. A retrospective audit of the haemodialysis population, the access performance and access management can be performed annually.

These audits identify individual and strategic issues, and initiate change. The audit of existing service provision allows areas for priority and for development, using national benchmarks.

Conclusions

The use of AV fistulae, grafts and CVCs for HD access varies considerably. Strategies to increase the use and longevity of AV fistulae for definitive haemodialysis access include vein preservation, early referral for access surgery, pre-operative clinical assessment of the venous and arterial systems, access surveillance, good cannulation technique, and aggressive intervention with surgical and/or radiological correction of AV access problems. The role of the VANS is diverse and challenging, but equally, is rewarding. The vascular access nurse specialist improves continuity and quality of care in these complicated patients, and helps to preserve vascular access longevity [12].

Key Summary

A VANS has an important role to:

◆ Ensure vein preservation.

◆ Ensure early and timely referral for haemodialysis access.

◆ Monitor the patient pathway for unforeseen bottlenecks.

◆ Maintain an advanced understanding of anatomy and physiology through comprehensive training to allow autonomy.

◆ Perform advanced clinical practice procedures, i.e. CVC insertion.

◆ Maintain a surveillance program of all existing access.

◆ Expedite failing access for intervention.

References

1. Tordoir JHM, Mickley V. European guidelines for vascular access: clinical algorithms on vascular access for haemodialysis. *EDTNA/ERCA J* 2003; 29: 131-6.

2. UK Renal Registry Report, 2005. Bristol, UK: UK Renal Registry. http://www.renalorg.com/report.

3. Report of Joint Working Party. The organisation and delivery of the vascular access service for maintenance. Haemodialysis patients (2006). www.kidney.org.uk.

4. Department of Health. National Service Framework for Renal Services, Part One, Dialysis and Transplantation. London: Department of Health, 2004.

5. Renal Association Clinical Practice Guidelines - Updates 2006. Vascular Access. www.renal.org.guidelines.

6. NKF-K/DOQI Guidelines. Clinical Practice Guidelines and Clinical Practice Recommendations: 2006 updates. http://www.kidney.org.uk.

7. Vanholder R. Vascular access: care and monitoring of function. *Nephrol Dial Transplant* 2001; 16: 1542-5.

8. Kumwenda MJ, O'Donoghue D. The changing options for managing blocked haemodialysis catheters. *British Journal of Renal Medicine* 2006; 11: 4.

9. Casey J, Davies J. Developing a nurse-led catheter insertion service. *British Journal of Renal Medicine* 2003; 8(2): 27-9.

10. Waterhouse D. Vascular access: a role for a renal nurse clinician. *EDTNA/ERCA J* 2002; 28: 64-9.

11. Konner K, Nonnast-Daniel B, Ritz E. The arteriovenous fistula. *J Am Soc Nephrol* 2003; 14: 1669-80.

12. Davidson IJA, Munschauer CE. The end-stage renal disease patient as related to dialysis. In: *Access for Dialysis: Surgical and Radiological Procedures*, 2nd edition. Davidson IJA. Landes Bioscience, 2002; Chapter 1: 1-10.

Chapter 18

The patient perspective

Stephen D'Souza MB ChB FRCP FRCR

Consultant Interventional Radiologist, Lancashire Teaching Hospitals, Lancashire, UK

Introduction

I first developed renal failure when I was 18, just after starting medical school, and have therefore been a patient longer than I have been a doctor.

Up until the time of writing this chapter I had never really considered quite how much my illness and experiences, as a patient, have affected my clinical practice. In hindsight, the areas that I, as part of a team, have striven to develop have paralleled the government thinking and recommendations, but were also based on how I would hope to be treated.

In recent years the UK government has introduced its healthcare modernisation agenda. Central to this is the concept of 'patient-centred care'. At the same time a number of other initiatives addressing the need for evidence-based medicine and accountability have been introduced. Whilst all these initiatives are intended to improve the delivery of healthcare, to some observers the desire to achieve one objective can have a negative impact on another.

Original experience as a dialysis patient

In early December 1982, I developed acute renal failure with malignant hypertension. At the time I was a first-year medical student with no clinical understanding of the situation. During that first two-week admission no one spoke to me directly about what had happened or its implications. Written patient information was not available in a simple understandable form and there was an unintentional tendency to confuse patients, by using medical terminology. As a result consent could not be considered fully informed and even when undergoing a renal biopsy only a minimal explanation was provided.

I was aware that I was quite ill but, for me, the uncertainty compounded the anxiety and with hindsight I had no real understanding of the consequences it would have in the future. There was a tendency for medical staff to gloss over issues or assume I understood more than I did.

The first time I was aware that I might need dialysis was when I was asked to sign the consent form for the creation of a dialysis fistula just before going down to the operating theatre. Although not required for three years, the timely creation of the fistula allowed it to mature before it was first used.

The first, informed discussion I had was some five weeks after my first admission, when I was admitted to a specialist renal unit. I will always be grateful to the registrar in renal medicine who spent a considerable amount of time explaining about my condition, in simple terms, and the likely prognosis. His task was made more difficult because he had to explain away all the mis-information I had received, from my main source of information, the other patients. It was only then that I appreciated the magnitude of the situation and that it would have an everlasting effect on my future. The most important thing he did was to make me be realistic about my predicament and take responsibility for the way I coped with the disease process.

In 1985, my condition deteriorated and I had to start on haemodialysis. I spent just over three years on haemodialysis, attending the unit three times a week. After the initial training, I felt it was important to be able to set up the machine and needle myself. This meant I was rarely delayed getting on or off dialysis and fortunately I have never had a problem with my fistula, which continues to work to this day.

During this period I was completing my medical training and starting as a junior doctor. My nephrologist considered "dialysis was a burden that should interfere with a patient's life as little as possible" rather than control it, unlike one of his colleagues. His support meant I could approach dialysis as a means to an end (i.e. transplantation) rather than an end in itself and in so doing continue with my medical career. Additional support came from the dialysis team and my colleagues at work without whose support I would have struggled to cope.

Apart from the time spent connecting and disconnecting from the machine and the dialysis itself, other time delays can make it difficult to lead a normal life. These include parking problems, delays with hospital transport, the need to attend separate clinic appointments and other hospital visits at other hospitals or on non-dialysis days, and mistakes with prescriptions. Although, on their own, these are minor frustrations and inconveniences, when added to the stress of the illness itself, it is easy to understand why small problems become such big issues. Sometimes it is easy for a patient to adopt the submissive role of an institutionalised patient, rather than struggle to maintain an independent life.

Coupled with the time limit, between each dialysis session, the geographic restrictions of haemodialysis are most evident when friends and family are planning short breaks and holidays. However, the opportunity for travel does exist. I was able to visit Jersey for a week thanks to The British Kidney Patients Association, who ran, and still run, holiday dialysis units in this country and Spain, but the most memorable trip was skiing in Bulgaria, taking with me a portable haemodialysis machine and some very supportive friends.

I received a cadaveric renal transplant in 1988 and although there were initial problems with acute tubular necrosis (ATN), the transplant functioned successfully for 14 years. Having been tied to the 'ball and chain' of my dialysis, this proved to be a very liberating time, although at the back of my mind there was always the concern that the transplant would eventually fail.

My renal function slowly deteriorated during 2002 and my care was transferred to the nephrologists at Preston. I started on continuous ambulatory peritoneal dialysis (CAPD) in 2003. Whilst still inconvenient, I find CAPD much less restrictive than haemodialysis and the introduction of erythropoietin means I have been able to work normally whilst on CAPD.

Providing arrangements are made in advance, PD fluid can be delivered anywhere in the world. I have been able to travel relatively freely with my most adventurous trip to date being to Florida, for two weeks. Thanks to the support of The Royal Society of Medicine, who accepts advanced delivery of the boxes of PD fluid, I am able to visit London without the need to take fluid with me.

I am now awaiting a second transplant.

Experience as a doctor

From my experience as a patient and a doctor, patients with a chronic disease process exhibit a range of responses from a passive acceptance of their situation, to a determination to maintain control as much as possible.

An expert patient task force was set up in late 1999 under the Chairmanship of the Chief Medical Officer, Professor Liam Donaldson, to recommend a new program that would bring together the valuable work of patient and clinical organisations in developing self-management initiatives. Task force members included representatives from the medical profession, non-governmental organisations, and experts in the fields of self-management training and research. The task force's report was published in September 2001 and included a key recommendation for NHS-based self-management training programs for patients [1].

Pilot Expert Patient Programme (EPP) courses began at 26 NHS Primary Care Trust (PCT) sites across England in May 2002, and by May 2004, approximately 300 PCTs had either actively implemented pilot courses or had committed to joining. The Department of Health sought to recruit a group of expert patients, who would be able to help guide future healthcare provision for chronic diseases [2]. The qualities they were looking for matched those of the patients who are able to maintain control:

◆   feel confident and in control of their lives;
◆   aim to manage their condition and its treatment in partnership with healthcare professionals;

- communicate effectively with professionals and are willing to share responsibility of treatment;
- are realistic about the impact of their disease on themselves and their family;
- use their skills and knowledge to lead full lives.

Helping the patient to maintain as much control as possible is an essential part of patient care, especially those with a chronic disease. Unfortunately, the NHS of the past has failed to support this group of patients and as a result created institutionalisation.

In 1996 I took up a post as Consultant Interventional Radiologist, at the Royal Preston Hospital. Since then the service has slowly developed and we now have a team of three interventional radiologists, four dedicated radiographers and seven radiology nurses.

My own experiences as a patient have been influential in the establishment of the interventional radiology service at Lancashire Teaching Hospitals and, in particular, the development of the vascular access service and more recently, the interventional radiology day unit.

As a tertiary centre for renal services I became involved in providing vascular access for dialysis patients, either by supporting the maintenance of functioning AV fistulae or by placing tunnelled central venous catheters (CVCs) when the nephrologists experienced complications or delays.

In order to address the problems of CVC placement, a staff grade nephrologist and renal nurse specialist were trained to place uncomplicated right-sided CVCs for haemodialysis, using ultrasound guidance. Check radiographs are used to identify any misplaced catheters and these are dealt with by the radiology team.

Initially, the radiologist-led CVC service was developed for the insertion of all left-sided and some complicated right-sided tunnelled CVCs, using ultrasound and fluoroscopic guidance in the radiology department. The change resulted in reduced numbers of complications and improved long-term patency of the catheters. This improved service and the development of a regional cancer centre at the Trust, led to an increased demand for CVCs, which could not be met by a radiologist-led service.

To address this problem a senior nurse and senior radiographer were invited to train to insert tunnelled central lines as independent practitioners. They now place the majority of CVCs used in oncology and nephrology. To reduce delays further, practitioner-led referral has been established. In oncology, the chemotherapy support team and PICC placers are able to request chest X-rays, line placements and removals without a clinician-signed request. Similar facilities are in place for the renal access team.

Naturally, CVCs are only used as a last resort for dialysis and the nephrologists, in the pre-dialysis clinics, and the two vascular surgeons, have made great strides to create AV fistulae in sufficient time to allow them to develop. As well as performing venograms and fistulograms, the interventional radiology services work to maintain vascular access. This is either through angioplasty and clearance of thrombosed fistulae or the use of alternative veins for tunnelled CVCs (e.g. femoral). One area that continues to be of concern is the lack of understanding some patients have of their fistula. From an interventional radiologist's point of view, most problems occur following an episode of dehydration and few patients understand the need to increase fluid intake in these situations. Better staff and patient education is needed to address this ongoing problem. Over the last three years, since the publication of the National Service Framework for renal services, the renal, vascular surgical and interventional radiology teams have attempted to provide timely vascular access which is monitored and maintained to achieve its maximum longevity [3]. Whilst there is still room for improvement this team approach is a significant improvement on the systems in place when I first started on dialysis.

Often patients are aware of my own personal experience and find it easier to tolerate the repeat visits some renal patients inevitably have to make to the interventional unit. Although I only tend to come across patients when they are having problems there is no doubt that good vascular access and a timely creation of an AV fistula are essential to a better prognosis. Occasionally the nephrologists ask me to speak with recently diagnosed patients. I try to encourage patients to maintain control of their care and be as realistic as possible about the future.

Joffe *et al*, amongst others, identified a number of factors that were influential in a patient's evaluation of hospitals, in which they had recently received treatment, and their perception of good care [4]:

◆ trust and confidence in providers;
◆ courtesy and availability of staff;
◆ respectful, dignified treatment;
◆ continuity of care and speed of transition;
◆ information and education;
◆ emotional support;
◆ inclusion of family and friends.

It is important to understand a patient's priorities and build up a rapport with them. As clinicians we tend to work on facts and figures; however, we need to recognise a patient's individuality and adapt our approach accordingly. There is a risk that staff will address those issues that they themselves perceive to be clinically important ahead of the patient's main concerns.

In the 1980s, one of the biggest problems I encountered was related to lack of patient information and staff education in this specialised area. Although specialist staff were called upon to provide advice, the information that was provided was not always consistent.

An example of this was when, before I started on dialysis, I was on a low potassium, low protein and low salt diet. The dietician provided me with three lists of food high in each and suggested that I should avoid everything on the lists. There was no suggestion about foods I could eat, just ones to avoid. The hospital catering itself was little better, reducing the total serving rather than reducing the foods to be avoided and increasing those that were allowed. As a result patients would become malnourished and well-meaning relatives would bring in extra, sometimes inappropriate, food. This is still a problem with the present day NHS.

On another occasion, whilst recovering from my transplant, I was regularly questioned about my reluctance to take my phosphate binding medication at the times prescribed (8am, 2pm and 10pm). It was clear some staff were uncertain as to their mode of action and therefore the reason for taking the tablets with food.

Sometimes the information was not available in a simple, understandable form and even when verbal or written explanations were provided the information could be too technical. Being a medical student there was a tendency to assume I had a greater knowledge and understanding than I did. As a result consent was not fully informed and occasionally procedures were undertaken without prior discussion.

Based on my own experience and a desire to provide a better quality of service for my patients, I felt that having access to our own beds was essential for development within the interventional radiology department. After a number of years of trying, the Interventional Radiology Day Unit opened in April 2006. It was designed to improve the quality of patient care, as well as improve the activity of the interventional radiology service as a whole by reducing waiting times and delays on the day of the procedure.

We try to provide a flexibility that fits in with the patient as much as possible. There are three pre-assessment clinics a week, led by two experienced specialist nurses and an advanced practitioner, and interventional procedures are undertaken five days a week. Sometimes, issues, unrelated to the procedure, but of concern to the patient, are identified and we attempt to address these or refer appropriately.

The pre-assessment visit can alleviate some of the patient's anxiety by simply introducing the patient and their relatives to various members of staff and showing them where they need to attend on the day of the procedure.

Patients are booked at appropriate intervals in order to maintain a calm atmosphere. The informed consent always includes a contact telephone number so that last-minute concerns can be addressed prior to the procedure and the consent is confirmed on the day of the procedure.

The unit has four beds and four reclining chairs. We attempt to maintain as much privacy as possible with curtaining and screens. The separate pre-assessment room is used for consenting. Patients are addressed according to their preference, which is established at their first visit. We encourage patients to bring a relative or friend to the pre-assessment visit and provide the latest up-to-date patient information (Royal College of Radiologists or National Institute for Clinical Excellence, if available) prior to obtaining consent.

The unit is also used to monitor in-patients in the first few hours following a procedure. Staff and patient concerns can be addressed promptly. In order to ensure good communication along a patient's journey, Trust-approved care pathways are used within the unit and between the unit and wards.

All patients are provided with contact details and a discharge summary, a copy of which is also sent to the GP. For all patients attending as day-case, a follow-up phone call is made the following day.

The essence of patient-centred care is to demonstrate a respect for the patient by addressing the issues that are important to them. It has been observed that "respectful care is unlikely to be perceived as thoughtless care" [5]. We believe our service has been able to achieve this. By trying to address the principles of patient-centred care we have created a service, which is more holistic and meets individual patient need, whilst improving activity and reducing patient delays.

My recent experience as a patient

My recent experience, as a patient, is that the nephrology service has improved significantly when compared to the one I knew in the '80s. At that time it was clear that whilst all the nephrologists were able to treat renal disease, only some could effectively manage a renal patient.

In today's NHS the widespread use of specialist nurses, working alongside nephrologists, who liaise with each other and provide consistent information, has helped greatly. The nephrology service is able to provide continuity of care that wasn't seen previously and in doing so reduces the 'institutionalisation' of renal patients. One potential downside of this new approach is that more practitioner/patient visits are required. As previously explained these visits can be on top of dialysis three times a week and its associated delays (parking, transport, faults with machines, access, waiting for drugs, etc). In order to minimise the patient's disturbance these visits can be performed at the patient's home or place of work.

In the majority of cases, the aim should be to re-establish as normal a life as possible once a patient receives a transplant. In order to do this, it is important that patients are given a realistic outlook from the time of diagnosis and are encouraged to remain as independent as possible.

It has long been suspected that some patients deliberately stop taking their immunosuppressive drugs as they are finding it difficult to cope with a life away from dialysis and its associated support and benefits. In the community there is a great deal of ignorance about transplants and their success. It is generally assumed that once a transplant has been performed the recipient is 'cured'. This misconception needs to be addressed, at a national level, so that an appropriate level of support can be provided. It is essential, for those more dependent patients, that the withdrawal of services is measured rather than sudden.

Conversely, those patients who are keen to 'get back to normal' should be aware that in the post-transplant stage, the status quo will be interrupted by hospital visits and their own concerns that any incidental illness is the first sign that the transplant is failing. There will also be concerns over the possible side effects of the immunosuppressants and other medication. Even if they are lucky enough to experience very few medical problems related to the transplant, their lives will continue to be affected by mundane issues such as life and travel insurance.

Overall, renal medicine, dialysis and transplantation have come a long way since I was first diagnosed. The ultimate aim of patient-centred care is to make coping with this life-long condition 'easier' for the patient; however, there are potential cost implications if this is to be achieved. A great number of changes have happened in that time but the one certainty is that it will continue to affect the rest of my life.

> ## Key Summary
>
> ◆ Always try to identify and address the patient's concerns.
>
> ◆ Ensure patient information is easy to understand and consistent.
>
> ◆ Encourage patients to lead as normal a life as possible.
>
> ◆ Keep hospital visits and patient inconvenience to a minimum.
>
> ◆ Create vascular access in a timely fashion.
>
> ◆ Monitor and maintain vascular access to achieve its maximum longevity.
>
> ◆ Try to be realistic about the future - it will never go away!

References

1. The expert patient: a new approach to chronic disease management for the 21st century. London: Department of Health, 2001.
2. National evaluation of expert patients programme: assessing the process of embedding EPP in the NHS: preliminary survey of PCT pilot. National Primary Care Research and Development Centre, 2004.
3. National Service Framework for renal services. London: Department of Health, 2004.
4. Joffe S, Manocchia M, Weeks JC, Cleary PD. What do patients value in their hospital care? An empirical perspective on autonomy centred bioethics. *J Med Ethics* 2003; 29: 103-8.
5. Baier A. Trust and its vulnerabilities. In: *Moral Prejudices*. Cambridge, MA: Harvard University Press, 1994: 130-51.